"Shawn Horn's book, *Thrive S...* date, neurobiologically based understanding of the emotional experience of living with ADHD, matched only by a master clinician's ability to bring the ideas and skills to life for readers to use. Horn's wisdom and compassion shine through as she guides adults with ADHD toward a new and better relationship with their emotions."

> —**J. Russell Ramsay, PhD, ABPP**, psychologist in
> independent practice, author of *Rethinking Adult ADHD* and
> *The Adult ADHD and Anxiety Workbook*, and coauthor of
> *The Adult ADHD Toolkit*

"Living with ADHD often brings feelings of shame, but it doesn't have to be this way. In *Thrive Socially with Adult ADHD*, discover how to transform your perspective, building self-compassion, acceptance, and interpersonal skills in ways that make life more manageable and fulfilling. This caring and practical guide offers invaluable support for anyone navigating the challenges of ADHD, empowering you to live better and feel like your best self."

> —**Mark Bertin, MD,** developmental pediatrician, author of
> *Mindful Parenting for ADHD*, and coauthor of *Mindfulness
> and Self Compassion for Teen ADHD*

"For many with ADHD, the most painful part isn't the distractibility and forgetfulness—it's the way it affects friendships and relationships. Just like with paying bills on time, ADHD makes it harder to do what you know in social situations. It also makes it easier for your emotions to get hijacked. Fortunately, *Thrive Socially with ADHD* offers you the tools to manage it all better. Your social life will improve, and so will your self-esteem."

> —**Ari Tuckman, PsyD**, international presenter, ADHD
> thought leader, and author of *The ADHD Productivity
> Manual*

"There's a painful void of books available to help adults with ADHD learn—in simple, clear ways—how our brain works and how it affects all aspects of our lives. Shawn Horn covers a lot of important ground, from taming shame to managing self-regulation and more. This engaging, sensitive guide combines science with practical, concrete, doable strategies. You'll walk away understanding more about your brain, your nervous system, and managing social situations (like how to remember people's names!)."

—**Terry Matlen, LMSW**, psychotherapist, author of *The Queen of Distraction*, and founder and director of ADDconsults

"Shawn Horn's book merges research on the brain and the nervous system with behavioral strategies to boost the social worlds of adults with ADHD. Themes of acceptance underscore practical, mindful strategies for managing symptoms. Readers will add this knowledge to their personal toolbox, while combating the negative self-talk and shame that can insidiously accompany ADHD."

—**Roberto Olivardia, PhD**, clinical psychologist and lecturer in the department of psychiatry at Harvard Medical School

"*Thrive Socially with Adult ADHD* offers a groundbreaking framework for transforming shame, rejection sensitivity, and emotional flooding into self-understanding and connection. Rooted in executive functioning science and polyvagal theory, this book introduces social executive functioning (SEF) to help adults with ADHD navigate relationships with more confidence and compassion. A must-read for anyone ready to rewrite their 'personal failing' story into a nervous system story—and to finally feel seen, understood, and empowered."

—**Lara Honos-Webb, PhD**, author of *Brain Hacks* and cofounder of ADHD startup, Bonding Health

"Although this book is intended to be a vital source of support for people with ADHD, it is actually a universal lifeline for all of us. Shawn Horn has tackled the most difficult topic in the world to write about—shame. It is the only emotion that does not seek expression. Even though everyone experiences shame, it is so primal and fundamental that it defies words. Horn has broken that barrier. She writes with beautiful clarity about the sources of shame and the personal experience of shame, and offers accessible and successful guidance about how to contend with feelings that we have never disclosed to another living soul. Be ready to be understood and helped in a way you never thought possible."

—**William W. Dodson, MD**, psychiatrist and internationally recognized ADHD expert

Thrive Socially
with Adult
ADHD

Shame-Busting Strategies
to Build Better Relationships Using
Polyvagal Theory & Neuroscience

SHAWN HORN, PSYD

New Harbinger Publications, Inc.

Publisher's Note

This publication is designed to provide accurate and authoritative information in regard to the subject matter covered. It is sold with the understanding that the publisher is not engaged in rendering psychological, financial, legal, or other professional services. If expert assistance or counseling is needed, the services of a competent professional should be sought.

NEW HARBINGER PUBLICATIONS is a registered trademark of New Harbinger Publications, Inc.

New Harbinger Publications is an employee-owned company.

Copyright © 2025 by Shawn C. Horn
New Harbinger Publications, Inc.
5720 Shattuck Avenue
Oakland, CA 94609
www.newharbinger.com

All Rights Reserved

Cover design by Amy Daniel

Acquired by Jenny Garibaldi

Edited by Joyce Wu

Library of Congress Cataloging-in-Publication Data on file

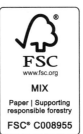

FSC
www.fsc.org
MIX
Paper | Supporting
responsible forestry
FSC® C008955

Printed in the United States of America

27   26   25

10   9   8   7   6   5   4   3   2   1   First Printing

In loving memory of my grandparents,
Carmen and Seymour Ratner.
Your words gave life to dreams.
Your love lit the way.
You helped make the impossible possible.
This is your legacy. I am forever grateful.
Love truly is the greatest gift.

Contents

Foreword

If you've ever walked away from a conversation feeling confused about what just happened—or worse, feeling like you were the problem—you're not alone. Many adults with ADHD experience social difficulties that aren't immediately obvious to others but that profoundly affect how they show up in the world. Over time, these experiences can lead to frustration, self-doubt, and a painful internal narrative: *What's wrong with me? Why can't I just get it right?*

Let me say this clearly: *There is nothing wrong with you.*

Social norms and expectations can feel opaque. Emotion regulation can be inconsistent. And the feedback we get—subtle and direct—can range from confusing to downright painful. We often feel like we're trying so hard, yet still falling short in ways we don't fully understand. It's not because we don't care—far from it. Many of us were never taught how to read the cues, calm our nervous systems, or interact from a grounded place of self-trust rather than shame.

That's precisely where this book comes in.

In this book, Dr. Shawn Horn brings together decades of clinical experience, a deep understanding of neuroscience, and her personal experiences to create a guide that feels both practical and profoundly human. She introduces us to the concept of social executive functioning—a framework that helps explain why things like conversation flow, tone, timing, and emotional responses can be so tricky for those of us with ADHD. And she does it without judgment.

This book doesn't tell you how to "fix" yourself. It helps you understand yourself. It offers a roadmap—not to being "normal," but to becoming authentically yourself. Dr. Horn provides tools for working with your brain instead of constantly fighting against it.

Drawing on polyvagal theory and the latest research in neurobiology, Dr. Horn helps us see how our nervous systems shape our social experiences. She teaches us how to notice when we're dysregulated, respond rather than react, and approach connection with more clarity and confidence. And perhaps most importantly, she gives us permission to show up as we are. Permission to release shame. Permission to stop apologizing for being wired differently—and start living with more intention, ease, and self-trust.

What sets this book apart isn't just the information it provides—it's how it's delivered. Dr. Horn writes with warmth and insight that makes you feel understood, not studied. Her voice is clear, compassionate, and refreshingly honest. She doesn't just share strategies; she walks alongside you as a guide. She knows this terrain from her training, work with clients, and lived experience.

Dr. Horn offers ways to navigate emotional overwhelm without shutting yourself down. She helps you understand why certain interactions leave you exhausted or confused. She equips you to enter social spaces more confidently, knowing you have tools and language that honor your neurodivergence.

Whether you are newly diagnosed, have been living with ADHD for decades, or love someone who is neurodivergent, this book will meet you where you are. It's equally useful for those seeking clarity and those seeking connection. It belongs on the shelf of every adult with ADHD— but more than that, it belongs in your hands, in your daily life, in the moments when you're wondering if anyone else gets what you're going through.

Dr. Horn has written a guide you can return to repeatedly—not just for the tools but for the sense of grounding and affirmation it provides. It's a reminder that you are not alone and that your struggles make sense. That change is possible—not by becoming someone else, but by becoming more fully and compassionately yourself.

Prepare to be seen. Prepare to grow. And prepare to finally feel at home in your own story.

—Stephanie Moulton Sarkis, PhD,
best-selling author and psychotherapist
www.stephaniesarkis.com

Introduction

Have you ever been told you talk too much? Maybe you interrupt without meaning to, overshare personal details, or struggle to keep emotions in check during heated conversations. Or perhaps you have a hard time reading the room, seeing things from someone else's perspective, or showing up on time to social engagements.

We've all been there—putting our foot in our mouth, cutting someone off mid-sentence, or accidentally breaking an unspoken social rule we didn't know existed. And let's face it, who hasn't experienced a bout of verbal diarrhea when nerves kick in?

For most people, these are occasional blunders. But for those of us with ADHD, they're not just occasional moments, they're just another Tuesday! What others might laugh off as a social hiccup, we painfully experience on repeat—leaving us confused, frustrated, misunderstood, and ashamed.

Do any of these sound familiar?

- Emotions hit hard and fast, making it tough to stay cool in heated moments.

- You replay conversations in your head, unsure if you said the "right" thing.

- You get so excited about a topic that you go full TED-Talk mode—before realizing *you've been the only one talking for twenty minutes.*

- You're nodding, engaged, and then—oh no! Did they just ask you a question?

- You genuinely *care* about people, but names, details, and key parts of conversations escape your brain like a pocket with a hole in it.

- You struggle to shift gears when a conversation suddenly changes direction.

- No matter how much you plan, five minutes can expand or vanish without warning. But when you're *in the zone*, you're unstoppable!

- When the people you love are out of sight, they're out of mind…until you remember them at 2 a.m., feel awful, and wonder if you should text them *right now*.

- You *want* to stay present, but your brain is like a browser with thirty-seven tabs open, and one of them just started playing music.

If you could relate to any of those, you're not alone. There's a reason it feels so familiar. Social interactions are complex for everyone, shaped by different backgrounds, expectations, and communication styles. But for us ADHDers, it can feel like trying to play a game where the rules keep changing and no one ever explained them to us in the first place. What seems intuitive to others is a trial-and-error process for us.

We may struggle to pick up on unspoken social rules, recognize subtle shifts in conversation, or manage the back-and-forth flow of dialogue. We may misjudge the right moment to speak, unintentionally interrupt, or say something that doesn't land well. Then, when our communication style clashes with social expectations, people may misinterpret us as selfish, arrogant, or disrespectful, even when that is far from the truth.

It's hard to even know what the "truth" is when we all have different experiences. We might walk away from an interaction riding the high of what we thought was a fantastic conversation, only to later learn that the other person walked away feeling the complete opposite. It's even more confusing when we receive mixed messages. One person might say we were the life of the party, while another says we're "draining to be around." How do we know which to believe?

And sometimes, we're perfectly fine until someone in our life tells us we're "too much." In the moment, we forget to even ask ourselves, *Who is saying this in the first place? Is their opinion credible or worth considering?* Feedback is subjective. Maybe you're not "too much." Maybe you're just too much for *that* person. Not everyone has the same capacity for high energy, enthusiasm, or depth, and that's okay. Their feedback reflects more about them than you.

All of these experiences of negative, conflicting, and unexamined feedback can leave you second-guessing yourself, constantly trying to decode what you did wrong (cue the sleepless nights replaying every conversation like an endless mental highlight reel). It can lead to a lifelong quest of asking, *Who do I need to be so that you're okay with me?*

The issue isn't *who you are*—it's that you've lacked the guidance, tools, accommodations, and insights ADHDers need to navigate these situations effectively. Without that support, misunderstandings grow, and isolation sets in. And when things aren't fully understood, they're too often met with shame, blame, and stigma.

Welcome to the journey of becoming a shame-buster!

Shame-Busters!

Shame and ADHD go hand in hand. From childhood onward, traits like impulsivity, emotional intensity, and forgetfulness were seen as misbehavior or laziness rather than expressions of a neurodevelopmental difference. Because of this, we were blamed for things outside our control, told we were doing things we weren't, and instructed to manage what we couldn't. Even when we gave it everything we had, we were still met with "try harder," "stop overreacting," or "be more responsible."

Our repeated failure to meet expectations led us to mistake neurobiological struggles for character flaws. When we could not measure up, we blamed ourselves. And when we could not change it, we shamed ourselves. Eventually, we began to believe maybe there really *is* something fundamentally wrong with us. That is how shame takes root. That is internalized shame.

This shame can continue to chip away at you, hijacking your thoughts, relationships, choices, and self-worth. And it can keep you stuck until you learn the truth about your brain, your nervous system, and your worth. For this reason, we must heal our shame wounds.

This is exactly why I've dedicated my career as "The Shame-Busting Psychologist" to help you break free from the grip of toxic shame—the kind that seeps into your identity and makes you believe you're broken, when really, you're beautifully unique with your own mix of strengths and weaknesses. Toxic shame doesn't belong in your story. It was placed there by a world that misunderstood your uniqueness and expected you to perform like everyone else. But really, who wants to be like everyone else anyway?

As a shame-buster, you see the value in your wiring and celebrate it. You meet yourself where you are, honoring both your strengths and your struggles. You know that being human means making mistakes, and that mistakes aren't something to avoid, but something to grow through. You understand that being human is messy, and life is messy. But messy can be honest. Messy can be beautiful. Messy is where growth happens.

This book is here to help you untangle shame from your story and your nervous system, so you can grow self-acceptance, compassion, and confidence. When you understand how your ADHD works, you can stop spiraling into shame and start living with clarity and connection.

The shame-buster approach is about honoring your individuality, embracing your strengths, and building strategies that actually work for your brain. Through insights and neuroscience, you'll come to understand ADHD as an executive functioning impairment and learn what accommodations you need to achieve what you're truly capable of. You'll also discover the missing link to social success: social executive functioning. These are the skills that unlock your ability to thrive in relationships and navigate the social world with greater ease.

Many will say, "I don't want to know why—I want the solution!" But understanding *is* part of the solution. It's the first step toward meaningful change. Because once you see what's really been going on, you can stop blaming and shaming yourself and start giving yourself what you've needed all along.

Before we dive in, let's get clear on what ADHD is and what it's not.

What Is ADHD?

The term attention-deficit/hyperactivity disorder (ADHD) is misleading. ADHD isn't a lack of attention—it's a difficulty regulating *where* attention goes. People with ADHD often experience misdirected or inconsistent attention; they might struggle to focus on things that feel boring or repetitive yet can hyperfocus intensely on something that interests them. It's not an attention deficit—it's an attention *regulation* problem.

ADHD is better understood as a neurodevelopmental condition of self-regulation and impairment in executive functioning. Let's break it down.

The term *neuro* refers to the brain and nervous system, which are both shaped by genetics and environmental factors. Genetics is the blueprint. ADHD is highly heritable and runs in families. The environment shapes how that blueprint gets expressed. Factors like stress, trauma, nutrition, parenting style, education, access to support, or even social expectations can influence how strongly ADHD shows up, how manageable it feels, and how much it impacts your daily life. So although you're born with ADHD, the way it plays out in your thoughts, emotions, and behavior is influenced by your life experiences.

The term *developmental* means it's present from birth and evolves throughout life, affecting how you manage attention, emotions, and behavior at different stages of life. Some people find that their symptoms improve with maturity, supportive environments, and treatment. For others, symptoms may worsen or resurface during key transitions, like hormonal shifts, increased demands at work or home, or the natural changes that come with aging. ADHD isn't static. It flexes and expresses itself differently throughout your lifetime.

Now let's look at the regulation piece.
ADHD involves dysregulation across the board:

- *Emotional dysregulation*, leading to strong, often overwhelming reactions like frustration, anger, or excitement

- *Behavioral dysregulation*, showing up as impulsivity, poor follow-through, or difficulty sticking with long-term goals

- *Nervous system dysregulation*, making it harder to stay calm, manage stress, and access executive functions

This is exactly why regulation is at the core of understanding and managing ADHD.

And this brings us to one of the most impacted areas: executive functioning. ADHD involves executive function impairments, which disrupt our ability to use these tools effectively—especially under stress or pressure. Executive functions cover a range of skills, and challenges can show up in different ways, such as:

- Working memory—keeping track of details and recalling information in the moment

- Emotion regulation—managing feelings without becoming overwhelmed or reactive

- Time management—sensing time, planning effectively, and following through

- Flexibility—adjusting to changes and shifting focus when needed

- Planning and organization—structuring ideas and completing tasks

- Decision-making—weighing options and making choices without getting stuck

- Impulse control—pausing before acting, speaking, or reacting

- Self-awareness—noticing behavior patterns and understanding their impact

Executive function impairments aren't about intelligence or effort. In fact, ADHD has nothing to do with intelligence; it is a disorder of performance, not knowledge. You may know what to do, but still struggle to do it. That's because executive functions bridge the gap between intention and action. When they're dysregulated, even simple tasks can feel overwhelming or impossible to start.

Executive functions also shape how we interact with others, a set of skills known as social executive functioning (SEF). SEF involves the cognitive, emotional, and behavioral skills that help you navigate social situations effectively. SEF skills help you follow a conversation, remember what was said, or stop yourself from oversharing. In short, it's executive functioning—*with other people.*

SEF is the foundation for all social skills. Without it, things like picking up cues, regulating your tone, or knowing when to speak can feel overwhelming or even impossible. Take remembering names, for example. Technically, yes, it's a social skill. But if your working memory is spotty, remembering names isn't just hard, it's heroic! So while name recall sounds like a simple polite gesture, for an ADHDer, it's more like a neurological magic trick.

This is where SEF comes into play. When you build SEF skills that work with your brain's unique wiring, you create the foundation that makes it possible to apply your social skills in real life.

As we explore ADHD, let's avoid a common trap: letting the challenges overshadow the strengths. Living well with ADHD starts by reframing the narrative to include what's possible. When we move from shame to a balanced view of both struggle and strength, we begin to unlock the full potential of our unique wiring and finally achieve what we're truly capable of.

Shame-Free ADHD

Learning about your ADHD is an invitation to explore your strengths and potential. The very traits that challenge you can also be the source of your greatest strengths and unique abilities. For example, impulsiveness might be the reason you took a bold risk that paid off.

Here are just a few ADHD strengths:

- Creativity—you think outside the box, bringing fresh perspectives to conversations

- Enthusiasm—your energy is contagious, making interactions lively and fun

- Emotional depth—you feel deeply and connect in meaningful ways

- Intuition—you sense emotions and shifts in moods that others miss

- Passion—when you care, you care hard; you go all in, and people feel it

- Resilience—despite setbacks, you keep learning, growing, and trying again

A strength-based lens helps you to see how your ADHD makes you extraordinary. The key is learning to harness the strengths of your traits while building strategies to manage the challenges. This book will help you do both, giving you the tools to regulate your nervous system, strengthen your SEF, and approach social interactions more effectively.

As an adult with ADHD and a psychologist with three decades' experience working with neurodivergent individuals, I deeply understand your experiences. I see you. I get you. I recognize your desire to decode the mysteries of executive functioning and to acquire the skills needed to thrive socially.

You might be thinking, *Just give me the damn instructions!*

Okay! That's exactly what this book is here to do. Unlike other ADHD books, this one focuses specifically on the connection between nervous system regulation and social-emotional functioning. It blends neuroscience, polyvagal theory, and evidence-based strategies to help you regulate your system, strengthen your SEF, and thrive socially with ADHD.

Who This Book Is For

This book is tailored for those who struggle with social regulation. Whether you've been formally diagnosed with ADHD, relate to these challenges, or support someone who does, it offers insights and tools to improve nervous system regulation and strengthen connection, communication, and understanding.

How to Use This Book

This shame-free guide breaks down both the "what" and the "how" of ADHD-related social challenges, turning knowledge into practical, actionable strategies.

In chapter 1, we start by building the foundation for learning: a shame-free growth mindset. Shame reinforces a fixed mindset: the belief that struggle means failure and that change is out of reach. But neuroscience tells a different story. Our brains are capable of growth and adaptation throughout life. A growth mindset supports this by encouraging resilience, experimentation, and self-compassion. It helps you see struggle as part of learning, not a reflection of your worth. When shame is removed, learning becomes easier, strategies stick better, and meaningful change can happen.

Next, we explore polyvagal theory and the neuroscience behind ADHD. In chapters 2 and 3, you'll learn how your nervous system is shaped by social interactions, relationships, and your sense of safety or danger. Understanding how your brain responds to stress and connection, and applying polyvagal-informed strategies, will help you regulate your nervous system, reframe your experiences, and strengthen your emotion regulation and SEF skills.

Chapters 4 through 9 focus on specific SEF skills, with practical examples and ADHD-friendly strategies. These aren't generic social-skills tips. They're foundational tools designed to help you use what you learn in ways that actually make sense for how your brain works.

Chapter 10 is all about reclaiming your voice and stepping into self-leadership. This chapter guides you in setting healthy boundaries, challenging internalized shame, and rewriting the story you have been told about who you are. It is an invitation to live shame free with ADHD, confidently, authentically, and in alignment with your values.

You can also find additional resources for this book at the publisher's website: http://www.newharbinger.com/56166.

What to Expect

As you move through this book, some strategies may resonate while others don't quite fit—and that's okay. There's no one-size-fits-all solution. Each person experiences challenges in their own way and to varying degrees. The key is exploring what works best for you.

Go at your own pace. Let the ideas settle. Talk about them. Try them. Revisit them. Many people flip through workbooks hoping for a quick fix, trying everything at once and feeling discouraged when results don't come right away. That familiar inner voice chimes in: *See? This doesn't work. Nothing works.*

But real growth takes time. Learning to regulate your nervous system, shift patterns, and relate to others differently is like learning to drive. Reading the manual gives you knowledge, but practice is what builds skill. At first, it's awkward. Then it clicks. Eventually, it becomes second nature.

The more you practice these strategies in daily life, the more naturally they'll begin to show up. Progress might feel slow, but it's still progress.

If you hit setbacks, it doesn't mean you've failed. It means you're still learning. Growth includes missteps. What changes over time isn't that the hard parts disappear, but that they show up less often, feel less intense, and are easier to recover from. Growth is about returning, re-centering, and practicing what you've learned. Your effort matters. Every stumble is a step forward.

Conclusion

By the end of this journey, you'll have a clear understanding of how ADHD shapes your nervous system, emotions, and social interactions. You'll gain practical tools to strengthen your social skills, regulate your emotions, and build more meaningful connections. Instead of feeling lost in conversations, overwhelmed by relationships, or hijacked by your nervous system, you'll know how to regulate yourself so you can thrive socially.

Most importantly you'll walk away with a shame-free mindset and strategies that help you lead your life in a way that aligns with who you are—not who the world told you to be.

Let this book be a source of clarity, empowerment, and renewed confidence in your social world. As you strengthen your SEF skills, trust the process. Take effective action. Know that each step forward, no matter how small, moves you closer to lasting growth and resilience.

Struggles will still happen, but they don't define you. Progress is movement forward, not perfection. It's about making mistakes, learning from them, falling down, getting back up, dusting yourself off, looking ahead, and returning to yourself again and again with compassion, wisdom, and courage. And remember this:

You're not behind.

You're becoming.

And you are perfectly imperfect.

Chapter 1

Shame-Buster

In classic ADHD fashion, we're diving in deep, right from the start.

You've probably heard the saying "Whether you think you can or you can't, you're right." That's because your beliefs shape your reality. They can either empower you to move forward or convince you to hold back.

One of the surprising perks of ADHD is that we don't always stop to calculate risk the way others do. Sometimes, we believe something is possible simply because we haven't paused to doubt it yet. That kind of boldness can be a gift. It's why we launch big ideas, take creative risks, and jump into things others might second-guess or overthink.

But there's one thing that can poison your beliefs, stop you in your tracks, push you into isolation, and convince you the possible is impossible—*toxic shame*.

If you read this book through the lens of toxic shame, looking for evidence to reinforce self-criticism, it can block your ability to learn, grow, and reach your goals. That is why this chapter is here: to help you develop a shame-free mindset, one that supports your growth, nurtures self-compassion, and empowers you to navigate challenges without self-blame and shame.

In this chapter, you'll learn:

- How shame manifests in your life

- The difference between a shame-bound and a shame-free mindset

- Three core skills to release toxic shame, build resilience, and embrace growth as a lifelong process

By transforming how you see yourself and your struggles, you will set the foundation for true change without the weight of shame holding you back.

Shame 101

Shame is a universal social emotion hardwired into you to ensure your survival. For your distant ancestors, being rejected by the group meant losing access to food, safety, resources, and protection, which could have been life-threatening. This is why shame is instinctual, fast, and intense, deeply linked to your survival fears. Its purpose is to signal when your behavior may jeopardize your connection with others, helping you stay in line with group expectations and avoid isolation or rejection.

But not all shame is the same; let's break down the different types of shame to understand this better.

Primordial shame: An autonomic nervous system response—like an involuntary reflex—triggered by a perceived social threat (*Freeze!* or *Something's wrong!*). It activates before your thinking brain can catch up. This physiological reaction has been observed in infants as young as fifteen months (Lewis 1995, 2022).

Healthy shame: A social correction, felt when you violate someone else's standards or expectations. It helps guide behavior and fosters learning (*Don't do that bad thing, or else!*). Healthy shame guides self-awareness, moral development, and empathy by steering behavior toward social appropriateness.

Guilt: An inner conviction felt when you violate your own values, principles, or standards. It motivates accountability and repair (*I shouldn't have done that "bad" thing*). Guilt, tied to cognitive development, emerges between ages three and six (Lewis 2022).

Toxic shame: When shame moves from social correction to identity condemnation, it becomes toxic. This is the deceptive message that you're fundamentally bad, defective, and unworthy *because* you violated someone else's standards or didn't meet their expectations (*You're bad because you did that bad thing* or *You're a failure*).

Internalized shame: Shame that takes root when you agree with the toxic shame message and now believe the negative messages you received (*I agree, I'm bad...broken...not enough*). Instead of feeling bad about something you did, you start to feel bad about *who you are.*

Shame-bound identity: The long-term result of internalized shame, where shame becomes the lens through which you see yourself and the world. It turns into a core belief about who you are and what you can expect from yourself—both now and in the future (*See! I will* always *be bad!* and worse, *That's how others see me too!*).

Rejection Sensitive Dysphoria

Rejection sensitive dysphoria (RSD) occurs when shame is triggered, causing overwhelming emotional reactions. Psychiatrist Dr. William W. Dodson (2019), an expert in ADHD, coined the term to describe a pattern he observed in his ADHD patients, who often experienced extreme sensitivity to perceived rejection, criticism, or disappointment from others.

Expressions of RSD include:

- Intense emotional pain from perceived rejection, even from minor cues like a short text or neutral expression

- Sudden mood shifts, where emotions swing quickly and unexpectedly

- Fear of disapproval or failure, constantly scanning for signs of rejection

- Emotional outbursts or withdrawal, with some reacting in anger or tears, and others retreating

- Persistent self-criticism, with negative thoughts like *I'm a failure* or *I'm too much*

- Perfectionism or people-pleasing, trying to avoid disapproval by overachieving or accommodating others

- Difficulty recovering from rejection, with the emotional aftermath lasting longer than the event itself

Although not formally recognized in the *Diagnostic and Statistical Manual of Mental Disorders* (APA 2022), RSD is widely discussed in ADHD communities due to its prevalence and significant impact on emotion regulation and social well-being. It is also not exclusive to ADHD. RSD can occur in anyone who has experienced repeated shame-based trauma, particularly in relationships where rejection or criticism threatened one's sense of worth.

RSD is a full-body trauma response, often shaped by chronic disruptions in connection that lead to interpersonal trauma. It's a deep, nervous system-level reaction to perceived threats and shame. So when your brain and body respond like it's life or death in response to social situations, it's not drama. It's not weakness. It's trauma—and it deserves care, not criticism.

Putting It All Together

Let's look at Johnny's story to see how these different kinds of shame presented in his life.

One day, Johnny went to the store with his mom and saw some candy he liked. Without thinking, he slipped it into his pocket to bring to his sister, who was home sick. At home, his mom found the candy while sorting laundry. "Johnny! What's this?" she exclaimed, her voice sharp with anger. Johnny froze, his body reacting instinctively before his mind could process what was happening (primordial shame).

"That's stealing!" she said firmly. The words stung, and Johnny felt terrible. She took him back to the store to return the candy, teaching him a lesson about right and wrong. Johnny thought, I better not do that again (healthy shame).

At the store, however, the owner pointed a finger and yelled, "You little thief! You're a bad boy!" (toxic shame). Johnny felt crushed. He hadn't realized that taking the candy was wrong. The harsh words left him ashamed and confused.

Later, Johnny found another piece of candy he had taken. Guilt washed over him: Oh no, that's stealing, and stealing is bad (healthy guilt). He confessed to his mom, who helped him return it and praised his honesty. Johnny felt relieved and promised himself to make better choices in the future.

But the story didn't end there. The store owner spread the word, and soon, parents warned their kids not to play with Johnny. He stopped getting invited to birthday parties. "You can't trust him," they'd say. Over time, Johnny believed the labels. I really am bad, he thought. I can't be trusted. This belief deepened into a sense of unworthiness (internalized shame).

As he grew older, Johnny avoided situations requiring trust, convinced he was destined to fail. To prove his worth, Johnny became a people-pleaser, but when he failed to meet other people's expectations, his inner critic reinforced his worst fears: I'll never be good enough (shame-bound mindset).

Even small critiques or rejections triggered overwhelming emotions. A neutral tone or missed "thank you" felt like undeniable proof that he was unlikable or a failure. These moments led to emotional outbursts, fueled by deep shame and fear of rejection (RSD). Each reaction only confirmed his belief that he was broken and unworthy (internalized shame).

Eventually, Johnny gave up trying. He apologized constantly, even when he'd done nothing wrong, and gave long-winded explanations to avoid criticism. Trapped in a shame-bound mindset and hypersensitive to rejection, Johnny lived on high alert—constantly bracing for judgment, convinced he would never be enough.

Becoming Shame-Bound

Toxic shame often starts in early childhood, when we're given the message that how we think, feel, or even who we *are* is wrong. These messages typically come from caregivers, authority figures, and peers. As children, we're especially vulnerable to shame because of its survival function and our dependence on others. Fitting in wasn't just important, it was essential for emotional and social well-being.

The cycle of shame is deeply embedded in families, often passed down unconsciously from one generation to the next. Because ADHD is genetic, many parents who struggled with it never received the understanding, support, or tools they needed to manage their own challenges. As a result, they may have been ill-equipped to meet the emotional and developmental needs of their children. Without the ability to regulate their own emotions, they may have struggled to provide the kind of attunement and support necessary for their children's nervous systems to develop a healthy sense of self-regulation and emotional resilience.

John Bradshaw (1988), in *Healing the Shame That Binds You*, describes shame-bound families as environments dominated by toxic shame, distorting the sense of worth for family members and perpetuating dysfunction across generations. In these families, unspoken rules suppress emotions and prioritize appearances over addressing real problems. For example:

- **Don't feel:** Emotions, especially negative ones, are suppressed to avoid conflict or judgment.

- **Don't talk:** Family issues are kept secret, and seeking external support is discouraged.

- **Don't trust:** Vulnerability is absent, fostering a culture of distrust.

- **Be perfect:** Family members must maintain an illusion of perfection to avoid criticism.

- **Keep secrets:** Transparency is avoided to preserve the facade of normalcy.

These rules leave children feeling unworthy and disconnected from their authentic selves. They are often expected to suppress their needs and emotions to meet impossible standards, becoming "perfect" to shield their parents from shame. This focus on appearances over solutions leaves children unprepared for adulthood while holding them to unrealistic expectations.

Toxic shame takes root in the shadow of impossible expectations, demands that can never be met. A child raised in a shame-bound family learns early that their worth depends on achieving the unattainable. Often burdened by their own unhealed shame, parents assign the child the rescuer role: *Be perfect so I can feel like a good parent.* When the child inevitably falls short, they believe *they* are inadequate and unworthy in a world of imagined perfection.

This weight becomes even heavier when the brain is wired differently, making success in a neurotypical world feel out of reach. Each failed attempt to meet expectations that ignore developmental differences deepens the sense of inadequacy. Instead of receiving guidance, they are met with disappointment, frustration, and rejection, creating fertile ground for toxic shame to grow. Over time, they stop believing they can succeed and start believing they *are a failure.*

Shame-Free Mindset

A shame-bound mindset is like carrying a relentless inner critic, always demanding more and telling you that you're not enough. It shapes your thoughts, emotions, and behaviors, often without your realizing it. Rooted in toxic shame, it distorts how you see yourself, how you regulate emotions, and how you connect with others.

But this mindset is not permanent. With awareness and effort, you can shift to a shame-free way of living, one that replaces self-judgment with self-compassion, fuels curiosity instead of criticism, and values growth over perfection. (There's a chart detailing the characteristics of a shame-bound vs. shame-free mindset at http://www.newharbinger.com/56166.)

The following three core skills can transform how you see yourself, connect with others, and navigate life. At first, putting them into practice may feel unnatural, but with time and consistency, they become second nature. So, stick with it—they work!

I can't tell you how many times I've had clients insist, "I can't do this. It's just not in my nature. I'm a judgmental person, and that's just how I am." My response is always the same: "Give it three months. Practice these skills, and I promise they'll start to feel automatic." And sure enough, three months later, they return surprised, saying, "It wasn't even hard! I just did it without thinking!" We both laugh, realizing they had hit that three-month mark right on cue.

That is the power of practice. As these skills take root, life starts to feel lighter. Relationships become easier, and connection feels more natural. When we let go of impossible expectations, both for ourselves and others, we make space for real connection, genuine appreciation, and a sense of peace we may not have thought possible.

Skill #1: Radical Acceptance and Effectiveness

Radical acceptance is the practice of fully acknowledging reality as it is—without judgment, denial, or resistance. It means accepting the facts of a situation, even when they're painful, frustrating, or unfair. It doesn't mean approval, agreement, or giving up. It means releasing the emotional exhaustion of fighting what's outside your control so you can focus on what *is* in your power.

This concept aligns with the wisdom of the Serenity Prayer: "Grant me the serenity to accept the things I cannot change, courage to change the things I can, and wisdom to know the difference."

When change *is* possible, the skill of effectiveness helps you take wise action. Instead of resisting reality or fixating on what *should* be, you focus on what *will work*, given the current situation. Effectiveness is about adaptability, practical problem-solving, and responding to life as it is—not how you wish it were.

The key principles of effectiveness are:

☑ **Work with reality.** Focus on what's possible, not what's ideal.

☑ **Drop the "shoulds."** Shift from "It shouldn't be this way" to "It *is* this way—now what?"

☑ **Do what helps—what will actually help—not what's fair.** Fair doesn't always fix it. Helpful and effective action does.

☑ **Adjust when needed.** If something isn't working, try something else.

Here's an example of how they work together:

You set a goal not to overshare at a gathering. But once you got there, excitement took over—and before you knew it, you were talking about your cousin's vasectomy, your weird mole, and the dream where you were dating a dolphin.

Radical acceptance says: *Yep, that happened. I got excited, and my brain went into storytelling overdrive. That doesn't mean I'm [fill in the self-criticism]. It just means I was dysregulated and doing my best in that moment.*

Instead of spiraling into shame or replaying it at 2 a.m., radical acceptance lets you name it without judgment—and move on.

Effectiveness says: *Given that it happened, what would help now?*

We'll go over tools for "what now" later. Until then, remember: It doesn't mean you failed. It means you're human—with an excitable brain and a good story (or ten).

Skill #2: Non-Judgment

Before we dive into the skill of non-judgment, it's important to know that judgment isn't the enemy. Judgment is a natural cognitive function that helps your brain categorize and make sense of the world. At its core, judgment is your brain identifying things as good or bad, right or wrong, safe or unsafe, familiar or unfamiliar. In its healthiest form, judgment becomes discernment, and discernment is essential. Judgment helps a teacher assess student progress, a doctor make a diagnosis, and a judge uphold justice. It also helps you decide whom to trust, where you feel safe, and what aligns with your values.

Judgments are also mental shorthand. For example:

- "Don't eat that, it's bad" might really mean "I left it out and it could make you sick."

- "That movie was terrible" might really mean "it's not my style—I prefer comedies."

The problem is that we often mistake these shortcuts as facts. And when others disagree, our brains may take it personally. You might think, *If they hated that movie I loved, they think I have bad taste!*—as if a different opinion equals a personal attack. That's where black-and-white thinking kicks in.

Black-and-white thinking is a hallmark of shame. It says you're either good or bad, a success or a failure, lovable or unlovable. It leaves no room for nuance or growth. This is why a judgmental mindset is often tied to a shame-bound identity. It creates rigid expectations, harsh self-talk, and emotional reactivity—none of which helps us grow.

Non-judgment, on the other hand, is about describing instead of labeling. It teaches you to observe your thoughts, feelings, and behaviors without attaching moral weight to them.

Instead of:

- *I'm so stupid for forgetting to call.*

- *She's terrible.*

Try:

- *I forgot to call, and that's frustrating. I'll call now to fix it.*

- *Her behavior is frustrating, and I prefer not to spend time with her.*

Here's the key shift:

- Judgment creates shame and inaction: *I'm bad. End of story.*

- Non-judgment creates insight and choice: *This happened. Now what?*

Non-judgment interrupts the shame spiral by replacing harsh labels with useful descriptions. That small shift makes a big difference—it gives you something to work with.

Over time, practicing non-judgment builds self-compassion and reduces emotional reactivity. You begin to see your experiences more clearly, respond more effectively, and move forward without dragging shame along for the ride.

TOOLBOX: Practicing Non-Judgment

Try these exercises to practice non-judgment:

- ☑ **Watch and describe:** Choose a reality TV show, news clip, or daily moment. Describe what's happening without judgment. Example: "The contestant forgot the lyrics," instead of "They're terrible at singing."

- ☑ **Reframe daily judgments:** Notice and reframe judgments throughout your day. Example: Replace *I'm so bad at this!* with *This is tough, but I'm figuring it out.*

Start small, stay patient, and watch how non-judgment transforms your mindset and approach to life. Let's now look at how this shift in mindset connects to the concept of personal culture and how it can reshape the way you interpret others' behavior.

Personal Culture

When we feel judged or misunderstood, it's easy to assume we've done something wrong. But often, we're just operating from different personal cultures.

Personal culture refers to the unspoken norms, habits, and expectations shaped by your upbringing, environment, or neurotype. Just like we wouldn't expect someone from another country to automatically know or follow our cultural norms, we can't expect others—even those we live with—to share all of our unspoken expectations.

What feels rude, confusing, or disappointing might actually be a mismatch in personal culture—not a personal failure.

Example:

Judgment: *They never text back. So rude!*

Reframe: *In my culture, fast replies show you care. In theirs, replying later might be totally normal.*

Judgment: *They acted cold and distant—I must have annoyed them.*

Reframe: *In their culture, quietness isn't rejection—it's how they process or recharge.*

This kind of culture clash can also show up in emotionally charged feedback:

"You're too much" might not mean you're inherently too intense. It might mean "your energy is more than I can process right now."

Reframing helps you turn criticism into insight—clues about someone else's preferences, limits, or needs. Instead of spiraling into shame, try:

- *Maybe I was talking faster than they could follow.*

- *Maybe they needed more quiet space or time to respond.*

When you stop hearing judgments as accusations and start hearing them as expressions of preference, it softens the blow. You can interpret feedback as *They're sharing what works for them* instead of *I'm doing something wrong.*

Remember—*Judgment loses its power when you stop taking it personally.*

Skill #3: Radical Self-Compassion

Self-compassion is the practice of treating yourself with the same kindness and understanding you would offer a good friend. According to researcher Kristin Neff (2011), it has three key components: mindfulness, which helps you acknowledge pain without exaggerating or ignoring it; common humanity, which reminds you that you're not alone in your struggles; and self-kindness, which encourages you to care for yourself instead of criticizing yourself when things go wrong.

But for those of us who carry deep shame, basic self-compassion may not be enough.

Enter *radical self-compassion*—a deeper, more courageous practice. Psychologist Tara Brach (2019) describes radical compassion as "a tenderness that arises when we are truly present and openhearted with our own suffering." It asks us not only to soften toward our pain but to turn toward it. To stay with it. To witness ourselves with full presence and care, even when we feel unworthy of love or afraid of what we'll find.

Radical self-compassion means being courageous in the face of your own vulnerability and shame. It means saying to yourself, *Even this part of me belongs.* You stop seeing your pain as something to hide, fix, or explain and start relating to it as something worthy of care.

Radical self-compassion is an act of strength; you face the very places that shame told you to avoid and meet them with gentleness, honesty, and humanity. It doesn't ignore mistakes; it reframes them as opportunities to learn and grow. It's not about giving up on change. It's about recognizing that you're perfectly imperfect and still worthy, even when you don't get it right. In showing up this way, you reclaim the parts of yourself that have been waiting to be seen and healed.

From Inner Critic to Inner Coach

Let's talk about your inner voice, the one that narrates your day. Is it kind or critical? Supportive or scolding? For many of us, especially those shaped by shame, the inner critic tends to run the show. But here's the twist: Your inner critic isn't trying to hurt you. It's actually trying to *protect* you.

The inner critic often emerges as a misguided protector. It tries to keep you safe by anticipating failure, rejection, or embarrassment before it happens, thinking that if it can shame you into avoiding risk, it can spare you from future shame. It believes that if you don't try, you can't fail. If you beat yourself up first, others won't get the chance.

But this strategy backfires. Instead of protecting you, it paralyzes you. It creates fear, self-doubt, and isolation. That's why it's time to introduce a new voice into the conversation: your *inner coach.*

Your inner coach speaks the language of radical self-compassion. It acknowledges mistakes without making them your identity. It helps you grow instead of shutting you down. The goal isn't to silence your inner critic. It's to thank it for trying to help, and gently redirect it:

Thank you for trying to keep me safe. I know you meant well. But I'm learning a new way now—one that leads with support, not shame.

Instead of seeing your inner critic as a bully to fight back against, view it as a part of you that's just doing its best with outdated tools. Then, step in with your inner coach and show it another way.

Here's how that shift might sound:

Inner Critical Voice	Inner Coach Response
You'll fail again—why bother?	*It's okay to feel scared. Let's try one small step and see what happens.*
Everyone else has it figured out but you.	*Everyone struggles. You're doing the best you can with what you know.*
You're so lazy—you can't finish anything.	*You're having a hard time focusing. Let's break it into smaller steps.*

You can reference this chart whenever you catch your inner critic taking the mic. With time, your inner coach becomes stronger and more automatic.

TOOLBOX: Kindsight

You can also build compassion with simple daily practices:

- ☑ **Kindsight over hindsight:** Instead of replaying mistakes with shame, reflect with compassion. Ask: *What can I learn from this?*

- ☑ **Name the pattern:** When you hear the critic, say, *Ah, this is the old protect-through-shame voice.* Naming it helps create distance.

- ☑ **Practice rewrites:** When a critical thought hits, rewrite it through the lens of your inner coach.

Radical self-compassion isn't a switch, it's a muscle. Some days it'll be stronger than others, but every time you choose a softer response, you're rewiring something powerful. You're building the kind of foundation that real change can grow from.

With time, your inner voice can become your biggest ally. That's the power of radical self-compassion.

And now that your inner coach is in your corner, let's take the next step: learning how to build shame resilience so you can live shame-free with ADHD!

Shame Resilience

Being shame-free doesn't mean you'll never feel shame again. It means shame no longer controls your narrative or defines your worth. A shame-free mindset shifts the question from *What's wrong with me?* to *What can I learn?* It creates space for growth, helps you stay grounded, and invites meaning from your struggles so you can learn from them—and celebrate your progress.

Shame resilience is the ability to recognize shame when it arises, tolerate its discomfort without letting it take over, and respond in a way that supports growth instead of self-judgment. Rather than defaulting to avoidance, perfectionism, people-pleasing, or self-criticism, you learn to pause, name what's happening, and choose a response rooted in compassion and your personal values.

Shame may still show up from time to time, but now, it's just a visitor. You don't have to invite it in, let it redecorate your mind, or hand over the keys. You can see it, greet it, and let it keep walking. That's what it means to live shame-resilient.

The shift begins—not when shame disappears, but when you stop living in reaction to shame and start responding from a place of self-trust, compassion, and conscious choice.

That's how shame loses its grip. That's how you reclaim your story. That's how you live shame-free.

Conclusion

The three core shame-free mindset skills—radical acceptance, non-judgment, and radical self-compassion—are not quick fixes. They are powerful practices that reshape how you think, feel, and respond. They help you meet challenges with greater clarity, intention, and care.

Building these skills takes time. When shame shows up, pause. Check in with your body, thoughts, and emotions. Understand what shame is communicating, then respond with care, not criticism.

There's no set pace or finish line. Growth isn't about becoming someone else, but becoming more of who you are—steadily, bravely, and fully. Your brain is wired for creativity, curiosity, and connection. Lean into those strengths. Whether you're just starting or deep in the work, it's never too late to grow.

You may never silence shame completely, and you do not need to. When delivered appropriately, healthy shame can guide empathy, learning, and repair. The work is to change your relationship with shame so it no longer defines your worth or directs your choices. You get to decide what stays, what heals, and what moves forward with you.

Chapter 2

Polyvagal Theory

What we don't understand, we shame and blame. When we don't know why we react the way we do, we make up stories to explain it. *I have no self-control! I always mess this up!* These shame-bound "you stories" (Dana 2018) turn struggles into personal failures.

But when you start understanding how your nervous system works, the "you stories" shift to nervous system stories. Instead of *I'm such a hothead!* you realize, *My nervous system gets overwhelmed in groups, making it harder to stay regulated.* This isn't an excuse, it's an *understanding*. And once you understand what's happening, you can actually do something about it.

That's where polyvagal theory comes in. Developed by Dr. Stephen Porges, it's like a user manual for your nervous system, except this one helps you make sense of yourself. By understanding your states, you can spot when your nervous system is shifting before you spiral into *Why am I like this?!* mode.

We'll do this using a traffic light model, a simple way to recognize whether you're in a green, yellow, or red state and, more importantly, what to do next (because let's be real—no one wants to stay stuck at a red light).

Fair warning, once you start seeing the world this way, you can't unsee it. You might find yourself diagnosing your friend mid-rant (*Oh, she's deep in yellow right now*) or realizing you are in red when you start rage-texting. As polyvagal expert Deb Dana says, "Once you understand the role of the autonomic nervous system in shaping our lives, you can never again not see the world through that lens" (2018).

Your Autonomic Nervous System

Your nervous system works behind the scenes to keep you alive and responsive. From controlling your breath to sensing danger, it adjusts unconsciously and automatically, shaping how you feel, act, and connect with others.

Dr. Stephen Porges's (2011) polyvagal theory revolutionized our understanding of the autonomic nervous system. He identified two distinct pathways of the vagus nerve: the *ventral vagal* branch, which supports safety, connection, and emotion regulation; and the *dorsal vagal* branch, which supports survival through shutdown and withdrawal. His theory showed that the nervous system isn't just about reacting to danger—it also adapts to promote connection and regulation when safety is detected.

Porges further theorized that the autonomic nervous system operates in three distinct states, each linked to different levels of evolutionary development. These states shape how you think, feel, and respond, and follow an evolutionary hierarchy. The newer systems that regulate connection (such as the social engagement system) support our well-being, while the older systems (like the fight-or-flight response) ensure our survival. Think of your nervous system like a house with three levels, each with its own function, supporting different aspects of your emotional and physical experiences:

- The top floor (ventral vagal)—the newest and most advanced system where you feel safe, open, and connected; where you experience social engagement

- The ground floor (sympathetic)—an older system that prepares you to take action when a threat appears; where you experience fight or flight

- The basement (dorsal vagal)—the oldest survival system, shutting everything down when escape isn't possible; where you freeze or withdraw in extreme stress

Your body moves between these floors depending on how safe or threatened you feel. When safe, you stay upstairs, interacting freely.

When stress hits, you move to the ground floor, ready to fight or flee. If danger feels overwhelming, you retreat to the basement, freezing to conserve energy.

This automatic process explains why you don't just think your way into feeling calm or connected. Your nervous system has to *feel* safe and connected. Your nervous system prioritizes safety, triggering automatic defenses beyond your control. These instinctive responses come from its oldest parts and take over when survival feels at stake, even if they override logic or social connection.

During a couples therapy session, I witnessed a surprising event that underscored the importance of understanding the nervous system. While the wife expressed her hurt and anger toward her husband, he suddenly fell asleep. I couldn't believe my eyes! He was alert and engaged just moments earlier, but as her emotions escalated, he seemed to shut down completely.

It wasn't because he had narcolepsy or didn't care; it was because his nervous system became overwhelmed. When his fight-or-flight response wasn't enough to manage the situation, his dorsal vagal shutdown response took over, causing him to disconnect and check out.

This example highlights how our nervous system unconsciously decides which state to activate based on perceived safety or danger. Understanding this changes everything. Without this knowledge, reactions to stress can be misinterpreted, which lead to misunderstanding.

But how does your nervous system make these split-second decisions without your even realizing it? That is where *neuroception* comes in. Neuroception is your body's built-in security system. It constantly scans your body, environment, and social cues to determine if you're safe, under threat, or in extreme danger, without conscious awareness.

Think of neuroception like a highly trained service dog. These dogs pick up on subtle changes—like shifts in cortisol, brain activity, or body language—often nudging their handler before the person is even aware something's off. Before my TEDx Talk, my coach's service dog leaned against my legs out of nowhere. I asked what was happening, and she said, "Looks like you needed grounding!" Sure enough, the dog had sensed my nervous system ramping up and calmed me with deep pressure—before I even realized I was anxious. That's your neuroception at work! It scans and detects signs of safety or danger, then cues your nervous system to bring the energy necessary to effectively manage the experience—like mobilizing to act, shutting down to protect, or staying calm and engaged. Let's take a closer look.

Nervous System States

Using a traffic light analogy, we'll explore each state and how it specifically influences your emotions, behaviors, thoughts, and body to help you recognize it in yourself.

The Green Light

The *ventral vagal* (*social engagement*) state is your green light. This is where you feel calm, connected, and engaged with the world. It's powered by the ventral vagus nerve, which sends all-clear signals throughout your body from areas like your throat, face, eyes, and ears.

In this state, your social superpowers activate. You can bond, communicate, and thrive in relationships. This is why it's called the social engagement system; it forms the foundation for connection, emotional resilience, and creativity.

When you're in a ventral vagal, green-light state, your nervous system is broadcasting safety and your whole being responds in kind. Here's what the green-light state might look and feel like:

Emotionally: You may feel calm, safe, and grounded. There's a sense of emotional steadiness, and you're more able to experience joy, connection, and contentment.

Behaviorally: You tend to be socially open and engaged. It's easier to stay present in conversations, enjoy time with others, and regulate your impulses.

Cognitively: Your executive functioning operates at its best. Focus and attention come more easily, memory improves, and creative or big-picture thinking is accessible.

Physiologically: Muscles relax, breathing slows, and your heart rate steadies. Digestion improves, sleep deepens, and your immune function strengthens. Your face is expressive, your voice warm, and eye contact feels natural.

What anchors it: Trusted social connections, shared laughter, time with pets, being in nature, or activities like singing, humming, or gentle movement—these are all ventral anchors that help you stay grounded and connected..

Imaginary road trip: Imagine cruising down the road with one of your favorite people. You feel relaxed and content, taking in the scenery and enjoying the conversation. Your gas tank is full, your car runs smoothly, and every traffic light is green. There's no rush, and you're in tune with your body, noticing when you're hungry or need a break. You pause to take pictures of the beautiful sights along the way. When you step out of the car, your body feels refreshed and energized. These are the kinds of drives you'll treasure.

Detecting the Green Light

To recognize when you're in a green-light state, ask yourself:

- *Do I feel calm, relaxed, and balanced?*

- *Do I enjoy being around others and feel present in my body?*

- *Am I aware of my body's signals for hunger, rest, and movement?*

Next, think about what anchors your green light:

- **Events:** *What experiences make me feel safe and connected?*

- **Situations:** *Are there places or scenarios where I feel most relaxed and open?*

- **People:** *Who helps me feel at ease and engaged?*

By identifying your green-light anchors, you can intentionally create moments in your life that support this state, helping you to strengthen and sustain it.

TOOLBOX: Vagal Toning Exercises

Your ventral vagus nerve plays a key role in how well you recover from stress, connect with others, and feel emotionally balanced. Just like a muscle, it can be strengthened through regular use. The stronger it is, the easier it becomes to access calm, regulate emotions, and engage socially. This ability is known as vagal tone—your nervous system's capacity to return to safety and connection after stress.

A weaker vagal tone means it takes longer to bounce back. You might feel stuck in anxious, reactive, or disconnected states. This can make socializing exhausting, emotions overwhelming, and recovery from everyday stress feel harder than it should.

Because your ventral vagus nerve connects to your breath, voice, face, and heart, engaging in these areas helps build resilience. These simple, body-based practices are known as *vagal toning exercises*:

- ☑ **Breathing**—slow, deep breaths with long exhales signal safety

- ☑ **Vocalization**—humming, singing, or chanting stimulates the nerve

- ☑ **Facial engagement**—smiling and eye contact activate social connection pathways

- ☑ **Sensory stimulation**—warm water on your face, gentle movement, and time in nature promote relaxation

Think of these as workouts for your nervous system. Practicing them consistently helps make calm, connection, and emotional balance more accessible, especially when life gets chaotic. You can find even more exercise ideas in the online resources at http://www.newharbinger.com/56166.

If this green-light state feels out of reach, it may simply mean your body is spending more time in fight-or-flight (yellow) or shutdown (red) states. You're not doing it wrong—your system just needs support.

The Lime-Green Blended State (Green + Yellow)

You feel grounded but energized, playful, alert, and able to bounce back quickly. Stress is manageable and connection feels natural.

On the road trip: The lime-green blended state is that energized excitement as you set off—relaxed enough to enjoy it, with just enough buzz to feel alive.

The Yellow Light

When your nervous system senses danger, it shifts into the yellow light state—also known as the *sympathetic fight-or-flight response*. In this state, the hypothalamic-pituitary-adrenal axis springs into action, releasing a cascade of stress hormones including *adrenaline, norepinephrine,* and *cortisol.* These chemicals prepare you to act fast—boosting energy, sharpening focus, and prioritizing survival over connection or long-term planning.

Emotionally: You may feel anxious, worried, or panicked (flight) or frustrated, irritated, and angry (fight).

Behaviorally: You may act impulsively, rush through tasks, argue, snap at, or avoid others. Patience wears thin, and social demands feel overwhelming.

Cognitively: Your brain struggles with focus, memory, and flexibility. Emotional reasoning takes over, and everything feels urgent.

Physiologically: Heart rate and breathing speed up, muscles tighten, digestion slows, and senses become more reactive. Appetite may change, and sleep may be disrupted.

What can trigger it: Perceived threats, sudden changes, overstimulation (crowds, lights, sounds), relationship conflict, pressure, deadlines, physical discomfort.

Imaginary road trip: Imagine cruising along when your fuel light suddenly flashes on. You notice you're miles from the nearest gas station. Your brain shifts into hyperfocus, scanning signs and exits, and the once-relaxing music becomes background noise. Someone cuts you off, and rage flares. You grip the wheel tighter, speed up, and burn more fuel trying to make it in time.

While this state can feel overwhelming, not all stress is harmful. Sometimes, this sympathetic surge can fuel productivity, creativity, and motivation. Known as *eustress*, this "good stress" can help you rise to a challenge—like nailing a presentation, running a race, or channeling adrenaline into a high-pressure task. For many with ADHD, this is the sweet spot for performance: focused, energized, and ready for action.

But even good stress has a cost. After prolonged activation, your nervous system needs time to reset. Without enough recovery, you may crash—experiencing what's often called a *post-event hangover or vacation blues*. This is your nervous system's way of demanding rest and repair. Balancing high output with intentional recovery is essential for long-term resilience. When managed well, this state can be a powerful tool—but only when it's followed by rest, regulation, and renewal.

Detecting the Yellow Light

To recognize when you're in a yellow-light state, ask yourself:

- *Do I feel energized, focused, or in the zone?*

- *Am I racing through tasks with adrenaline-fueled momentum?*

- *Do I feel excited or driven, but maybe also a little wired?*

- *Am I juggling multiple thoughts or projects at once with intensity?*

If these sound familiar, you may be in the "buzz zone."

Positive answers to these next questions may indicate you're in "overdrive":

- *Do I feel stressed, rushed, or overwhelmed?*

- *Do I get easily frustrated, impatient, or reactive?*

- *Are noises, interruptions, or social demands starting to feel irritating?*

- *Do I feel socially avoidant or overstimulated by people?*

- *Is it hard to slow down, fall asleep, or truly relax?*

Next, think about what triggers your yellow light:

- **Events:** *What situations make me feel stressed or on edge?*

- **Places:** *Are there environments where I feel particularly tense or overstimulated?*

- **People:** *Who tends to provoke a fight-or-flight response in me?*

TOOLBOX: Regulating the Yellow

When your yellow light kicks in, your body floods with adrenaline and cortisol, revving up your system for action. That surge of stress hormones creates a buildup of energy and tension in the body—energy that needs to be used or released. If it stays stuck, it can lead to overwhelm, irritability, or burnout. The goal is to discharge that energy, calm the nervous system, and anchor yourself back to ventral so you can think clearly and respond intentionally.

Try these activities to regulate your yellow-light state:

☑ **Move to discharge energy.** Burn off excess adrenaline and cortisol through physical activity to help your body reset:

- Take a brisk walk, run, or stretch.
- Dance to a favorite song or try yoga.
- Practice progressive muscle relaxation (tense and release muscles).

☑ **Ground through your senses.** Use sensory input to anchor yourself in the present moment and calm your nervous system:

- Splash cold water on your face or hold an ice cube.
- Use calming scents like lavender or eucalyptus.
- Listen to soothing music or focus on calming sounds.

☑ **Express and release emotion.** Let the pressure out by giving your emotions somewhere to go:

- Write down your thoughts or emotions in a journal.
- Draw, paint, or engage in creative activities.
- Hum, sing, or breathe deeply to stimulate your vagus nerve.

☑ **Reassure and reset.** Remind your system that you're safe and in control:

- Try box breathing (inhale for 4 counts, hold for 4, exhale for 4, hold for 4).
- Use calming self-talk, like *I can manage this.*
- Focus on gratitude—name three things you're thankful for.

Blended Orange State (Yellow + Red)

You feel stuck and overwhelmed, but energy is still surging. This can lead to erratic or explosive reactions.

On the road trip: It's like running low on gas and snapping at your friend: "Stop talking! I can't focus!" You're frozen and frantic all at once.

The Red Light

When your nervous system reaches its breaking point, it shifts into the red light, your dorsal vagal (freeze, flop, or fawn) state. This full-body shutdown is governed by the dorsal vagus nerve, the oldest branch of the vagus system. It runs from your brainstem to organs below your diaphragm, including your stomach, intestines, and other systems involved in digestion and regulation. When this system activates, your body slows down, pulls inward, and shuts off nonessential functions so you can endure.

Think of it like the overflow drain in a bathtub. When stress floods your system, this response diverts the overflow, not to fix it, but to keep you from drowning. Just like a possum that instinctively goes limp when threatened, your body drops into stillness. Pain is muted, energy conserved, and awareness narrows to the bare minimum. This is a survival reflex, a biological way of saying, "There's no way out, so we're going into hibernation mode."

In this state, you may feel heavy, foggy, numb, or emotionally flat. It might seem like you've shut down or given up, but this isn't failure—it's your nervous system's last-ditch strategy when it senses there's no safe path forward. Your body says, "I can't fight, and I can't flee—so I'll freeze." Just like a possum that instinctively goes limp when threatened, your body drops into stillness. Pain is muted, energy is conserved, and awareness narrows to the bare minimum. This is your survival response.

Alongside this, your mind may disconnect from your experience in a process called *dissociation*. You might feel like you're floating outside your body, watching yourself from a distance, or like time has gone missing. You might catch yourself zoning out, unable to recall parts of a conversation, or feeling strangely numb and unreachable—even to yourself. As confusing or frustrating as that disconnection may feel, it's actually a protective buffer, giving your system space from sensations and emotions that would otherwise be too overwhelming to process in real time. There's a kind of ancient wisdom in this state that quietly says, "Let's survive this moment first. The rest can come later."

Emotionally: You may feel hopeless, numb, ashamed, or detached. Emotions seem distant or out of reach.

Behaviorally: You may withdraw, speak less, move slowly, or avoid connection. Basic tasks feel too heavy.

Cognitively: Executive functioning struggles. Time may distort, memory fades, and dissociation sets in—you feel spaced out, outside your body, or forgetful.

Physiologically: Breathing slows, heart rate drops, digestion stalls, and pain dulls. You may feel cold, disconnected, or experience chronic issues like fatigue, low blood pressure, or inflammation.

What can trigger it: Prolonged stress, trauma, shame, social rejection, burnout, exhaustion, illness, or unmet needs like food and sleep.

Imaginary road trip: On your imagined drive with friends, you approach a train track, and you can see that a long train is coming. You try to beat it but fail, and the light turns red, forcing you to stop. As the gate lowers in front of you and the train whizzes by, your car stalls. It's out of gas. Defeated and exhausted, you wish you could disappear. Thinking clearly feels impossible, and you're so disconnected that you don't notice your hunger or need to use the restroom. Lost in your thoughts, you zone out until your friend says, "Hello, are you there?" Snapping back, you mumble, "Oh, sorry, I must have checked out."

This protective buffer gives your system distance from sensations and emotions too overwhelming to process in real time. This is your body's ancient wisdom helping you endure the unendurable.

"Calm" in Crisis

"I've always been unusually calm in a crisis, with a high pain tolerance, low blood pressure, and heart rate. Nothing bothers me—I'm as
calm as calm can be!" Yet that same person also struggles with chronic
health issues like autoimmune conditions, inflammation, poor sleep, and
trouble managing stress.

In these cases, their body is signaling a chronic dorsal vagal state,
not stellar health or strong character. While these responses might seem
helpful in the short term, they can become a lasting state when the
nervous system stops expecting support and shuts down to protect itself.
It's a survival strategy, not a badge of honor. Recognizing this shift as a
protective mechanism is the first step toward real healing. So watch out
for low blood pressure and heart rate, high pain tolerance, and an unusual
calm when all of that doesn't make sense with your current state of
health.

Detecting the Red Light

To identify when you're in the red-light state, ask yourself:

- *Do I feel isolated, numb, or disconnected from others?*

- *Is it hard to stay focused and alert, or make decisions?*

- *Do I feel completely drained, with little energy or motivation?*

- *Do I handle emergencies with unusual calm, as if I'm detached
  from the situation?*

- *Do I have a high pain tolerance or experience physical symptoms
  like low heart rate or low blood pressure?*

Next, think about what activates your red light:

- **Events:** *Are there specific situations or experiences that leave
  me feeling overwhelmed or frozen?*

- **Settings:** *Are there environments that make me feel emotionally disconnected or withdrawn?*

- **People:** *Are there individuals who trigger feelings of shame, helplessness, or rejection?*

By identifying your triggers and recognizing the signs of your redlight state, you can begin to understand what causes you to shut down. Awareness is the first step in learning how to respond with compassion and care for yourself.

TOOLBOX: Gentle Reawakening

In the red-light state, your nervous system needs gentle, patient care to reawaken energy and reconnect to the world. Think of this as your "rest and recharge" zone. The goal is to help your system come back online slowly, without overwhelm.

Try these steps:

- ☑ **Gentle movement:** Start small. Stretch, stand up, or take a slow walk to ease your body into activity.

- ☑ **Safe connection:** Spend time with someone who feels grounding, whether it's sitting quietly with a trusted person or cuddling with a pet.

- ☑ **Focus on basics:** Break tasks into tiny steps, like sipping water or having a small snack, to rebuild energy.

- ☑ **Rebuild slowly:** Don't rush. Give yourself permission to take your time. Your nervous system needs time and space to recover.

Patience is key here. Small, consistent actions can help you gently shift out of shutdown and anchor yourself back to your ventral vagal state, allowing your system to complete the stress cycle.

The Blended Gray State (Red + Green)

You feel disconnected or spaced out but can still engage on the surface. You're functioning socially, but your body is in shutdown.

On the road trip: Think zoning out in the passenger seat, nodding along to conversation but not really present.

TOOLBOX: Run, Roar, or Rest

Now that you can recognize your nervous system (and in-between) states, the next step is knowing how to work with them. Different states call for different responses:

- **Run (Flight):** Anxious or jittery? Move—walk, dance, or stretch to release energy.

- **Roar (Fight):** Frustrated or on edge? Channel it—journal, vent, or create.

- **Rest (Freeze):** Numb or exhausted? Soothe—breathe, sip water, use gentle sensory input.

The more you match your actions to your state, the faster you'll regulate your state and build resilience.

Conclusion

There's a saying that the longest journey is from the head to the heart. That's because your thinking brain and ANS feeling brain don't speak the same language. Your ANS doesn't respond to logic, pep talks, or color-coded to-do lists. It responds to sensation, emotion, and energy. It listens to your breath, your posture, your tone of voice, and the rhythm of your day. Regulation isn't something you can think your way into. It's something you practice, feel, and embody. You can't outthink a dysregulated nervous system. You have to learn how to work with it.

Learning the language of your nervous system is like discovering a secret radio station you didn't know was playing in the background. At first, the signal is fuzzy. But the more you tune in, the more clearly you hear what your body is trying to say. With practice, you start to recognize the cues faster and respond more effectively. That helps you recover more quickly when life throws you off track.

You don't have to get it perfect. You just have to get curious and pay attention to what your body is broadcasting. That's how you become an expert state detector. You tune in, feel through, and respond to your needs. Understanding your nervous system helps bridge the gap between unconscious reaction and conscious response. It brings your body's automatic instincts into alignment with your brain's intentional awareness. When you can recognize and regulate your state, you stop being ruled by your reactions and start responding with regulated intention.

Next, we'll explore how this applies to the ADHD nervous system. You'll learn how neurodivergent brains interpret and respond to safety, connection, and threat differently from neurotypical ones, and most importantly, how you can harness your nervous system's unique wiring for greater well-being.

Chapter 3

ADHD Wiring

Consider this snapshot:

8 a.m. While the world is up and running, your brain feels like an old car that's been parked too long. After a few rounds of snoozing, you finally get moving, but the gears are sluggish. Just as you hit your stride by mid-morning, everyone else has already shifted into their next gear.

12 p.m. At lunch, coworkers chat about weekend plans. But the clinking dishes, the sound of chewing, the music, and Jordan's laugh (seriously, why is it so *loud*?) leave you drowning in sensory overload.

3 p.m. While everyone else's energy begins to crash, you're in the zone. Your brain is in overdrive, solving problems at lightning speed.

6 p.m. Happy hour sounds great. But first, you stop at home and...as you sit in the driveway, debating whether to go out, your brain makes the call—we're done. While others can rally, your engine shuts off completely.

10 p.m. Hello, ADHD second wind! Powered up and buzzing with ideas, you tackle that long-avoided project. By 3 a.m. you've accomplished a ton—except...sleeping.

Morning looms, and in five hours, *it all starts again!*

This is just one example of how our bodies are out of sync with the world around us. What's "normal" doesn't always apply to you, especially when it comes to your nervous system.

What *is* universal for ADHDers is that the unexpected is expected, the inconsistency is consistent. It's a wild, confusing ride.

This chapter dives into the asynchronistic nature of ADHD and helps you understand the unique ways your nervous system operates. You'll also learn specific tools to regulate each state more effectively.

Out of Sync

Have you ever felt like you're behind socially, emotionally, or even physically compared to others your age? Like you're always playing catch-up, no matter how hard you try? You're not imagining it.

Brains develop at their own pace, but most people hit common milestones, like walking and talking, around certain ages. Some may reach them sooner or later, and that's normal. Brain development happens in stages: first the lower regions for basic functions, then the mid-brain for emotions, and finally the prefrontal cortex, responsible for self-control, organization, and decision-making. This last part typically matures in neurotypical people by the mid-twenties.

The ADHD brain develops on a different timeline than neurotypical peers, with full maturation often extending into the late twenties or even thirties. This delay is largely due to two key factors: asynchronous development and what's known as the 30-percent rule.

Asynchronous development means that the brain doesn't develop in an even and predictable way. Some areas, like creativity or problem-solving, may mature faster, while others, like emotion regulation or impulse control, take longer. This uneven growth often makes ADHDers feel out of sync with peers and contributes to why many are seen as "late bloomers."

According to Dr. Russell Barkley's *30-percent rule* (2012), ADHDers typically experience a 30-percent delay in executive functions, emotion regulation, and social maturity compared to neurotypical peers.

In real-world terms:

- A ten-year-old with ADHD may have the emotion regulation of a seven-year-old

- A twenty-year-old may navigate social functions like a fourteen-year-old

This is why tasks and self-control felt more challenging than others—the prefrontal cortex needed more time to catch up.

Because of asynchronous development and this 30-percent delay, ADHDers often face gaps in skills like planning, impulse control, and organization. These gaps can lead to:

- **Inconsistent performance:** You might shine in some areas while struggling with everyday tasks.

- **Relationship challenges:** Social interactions may feel confusing, exhausting, or isolating.

- **Academic and work challenges:** Tasks like time management or meeting deadlines can be challenging.

This mismatch between your expectations and abilities can create chronic stress. You may feel like you're always trying to catch up, even when giving your best. As children, this confusion leads to frustration and shame. It's no wonder you felt out of sync or frustrated, especially when others seemed to meet milestones or expectations with ease. Your brain was simply catching up at its own pace, and that's okay!

Shame-buster reframe: Your brain developed at its own pace, and that's completely fine! The fact that you may have had a different rhythm doesn't make you any less capable—just give yourself the space and grace to catch up, on your own timeline.

Now let's look at differences in ADHD chemistry and stress responses.

ADHD, Cortisol, and the Stress Response

ADHD changes how your body handles stress, not just mentally but chemically. When something stressful happens, your body releases three key chemicals: adrenaline, norepinephrine, and cortisol. Adrenaline gives you a quick burst of energy. Norepinephrine sharpens your focus. Cortisol manages the whole process. It helps keep you alert and steady during longer stress, then steps in to calm your system when the stress is over.

Think of cortisol as the manager of your stress team. It keeps things from getting too intense, helps prevent emotional overload, and supports recovery afterward. It also plays a role in inflammation, immune function, and mental clarity. But in ADHD, this manager doesn't always show up on time or do its job well.

People often think the problem is having too much or too little cortisol. But in ADHD, the real issue is cortisol dysregulation. It's not just about the amount. It's about timing, rhythm, and balance. Cortisol might be too low when you need it, be too high when you need to wind down, or show up late. That can lead to:

- Feeling the effects of adrenaline and norepinephrine more intensely

- Stress that lasts longer in your body and mind

- A harder time bouncing back and feeling like yourself again

This makes emotional reactivity, post-stress crashes, and low resilience more common. This happens not because you're weak, but because your chemistry is out of sync.

Cortisol also follows a daily rhythm called the *diurnal rhythm*. It's supposed to rise in the morning to help you wake up and drop at night so you can relax and sleep. But for many of us, this rhythm is flipped. Cortisol is low in the morning, making it hard to get going, and high at night, making it hard to calm down. That can leave you foggy during the day and wired at bedtime.

So if you've ever wondered why stress hits harder, why emotions feel so intense, why mornings are rough, and why you get a second wind at bedtime—now you know. It's cortisol dysregulation in ADHD.

It all starts to make more sense. These chemical imbalances and dysregulation explain why life can feel so overwhelming and why it's easy to get stuck in the yellow and red zones.

Shame-buster reframe: It's not about willpower; it's about regulation!

I can hear your thought now—*Okay, but what do I do about it?*

Regulating cortisol, especially when it's too low, too high, or out of rhythm, starts with supporting your nervous system and reducing chronic stress. The good news is that lifestyle and behavioral changes can help improve its balance over time. For specific tips on regulating cortisol levels, visit the online resources at www.newharbinger.com/56166.

Now, let's dive into how this shows up in your nervous system, starting with the yellow zone, that familiar blend of urgency, emotional intensity, and hyperfocus. It comes with its own set of challenges and surprising strengths.

ADHD Yellow Light

While others get overwhelmed by intensity, this is where we come alive. Pressure fuels momentum, and urgency flips the switch. A looming deadline? Suddenly, you're unstoppable. A high-stakes challenge? Your brain fires on all cylinders, ideas flowing faster than you can catch them. In the yellow zone, everything feels urgent—and that urgency is what gets things done.

Of course, this energy has its quirks, such as overtalking (oversharing, interrupting, blurting), emotional intensity (a neutral comment triggering an emotional tidal wave), heightened sensitivity (a simple mistake feeling like a catastrophe), and losing time. The issue isn't just the quirks, but that our nervous system isn't built to "turn the volume down" easily. ADHD brains are wired for intensity, making it difficult to shift between calm and action.

Hyperfocus: The ADHD Spotlight Effect

Hyperfocus is one of ADHD's most misunderstood traits—sometimes a superpower, sometimes a trap. For us, focus isn't a dial; it's a switch—either off or blindingly bright, often flipped by urgency, stress, or pressure.

It can be a strength when you're in control, but when it takes over, it can derail your priorities. As you learned in the previous section, dopamine and norepinephrine regulate focus, motivation, and energy. When dopamine is high, it sharpens attention and filters distractions like a spotlight snapping on. When it's low, even simple tasks feel impossible. So the ADHD brain turns to stress hormones like adrenaline and cortisol as backup fuel.

That's why we depend on deadlines, last-minute pressure, and urgency to function. Stress becomes the motivator when dopamine isn't doing its job. Stress-driven hyperfocus feels like panic, and while it works temporarily, it's unsustainable. Over time, it keeps the nervous system stuck in yellow, a state of chronic stress and heightened arousal, making it hard to shift between states (Arnsten 2009; Porges 2011; Shaw et al. 2014). The yellow zone becomes your nervous system default. Life without urgency feels unnatural.

In yellow, stress and urgency fuel intense concentration. You're in the zone when:

- A deadline pushes you into beast mode

- A creative spark pulls you into flow

- A fast-paced job keeps you fully engaged

- A hyperfixation locks you in for hours

Hyperfocus feels powerful until it doesn't:

- You forget basic needs—eating, drinking, sleeping

- You look up and realize five hours have vanished (time blindness)

- You run on urgency until you crash (burnout loop)

- You deep-dive into a random rabbit hole, hyperfocusing on the wrong thing

TOOLBOX: Making Hyperfocus Work for You

Instead of waiting for panic to activate you into action:

☑ **Set time limits**—alarms or timers can snap you out of the vortex.

☑ **Plan deep work sessions**—give yourself structured hyper-focus time.

☑ **Listen to body signals**—hunger, exhaustion, or tension means it's time to step away.

☑ **Use accountability**—ask a friend to check in and pull you out when needed.

Neuroception Distortion: When Safety Feels Like Threat

As you just learned, cortisol dysregulation makes stress responses more intense and harder to shut off. That's why many adults with ADHD have nervous systems that activate more easily and stay stuck longer (Arnsten 2009). When this happens, your brain flips into survival mode, scanning for signs of danger. But instead of reading the room accurately, your nervous system distorts the picture—zooming in on anything that feels threatening and tuning out cues of safety (Porges 2011). This is called *neuroception distortion*.

ADHD brains are also wired to prioritize negative emotions, picking up on subtle signs of disapproval or rejection while overlooking neutral or positive cues (Shaw et al. 2014). This combination—heightened sensitivity and negative filtering—can make everyday moments feel emotionally loaded. For example:

- A neutral face looking angry or threatening because your brain amplifies tiny cues of disapproval

- A short reply, a delayed text, or an unread message feeling like rejection, triggering an emotional reaction before logic kicks in

- Background noise, overlapping conversations, or unexpected sounds becoming unbearable, making it harder to regulate emotions

When your perception is shaped by a dysregulated nervous system, it's easy to question your own reality later. You may find yourself wondering:

- *Was that actually rude, or was I just overwhelmed?*

- *Did they ignore me, or was I just anxious?*

- *Was I justified in feeling that way, or did I overreact?*

This cycle of doubting yourself after an emotional reaction is a form of self-gaslighting, where you invalidate your own experiences because you struggle to trust your perceptions. Over time, this can make you second-guess your instincts, needs, and even your own emotions.

We'll talk more about gaslighting in chapter 10. For now, let's move on to how to get out of a self-doubt loop.

TOOLBOX: The 24-Hour Rule

When emotions are running high, perception gets distorted—so it's best to "sober up" emotionally before making decisions. One of the most effective ways to do that is the 24-hour rule: wait a full day before reacting, especially if you feel triggered. No angry texts, quitting on impulse, or jumping to conclusions.

Instead, regulate first by stepping away, breathing, moving your body, or talking to a trusted person. Once your nervous system settles, reassess:

- *Does this still feel like a big deal?*

- *Was I activated, or is this something I need to address?*

For most people, a day is enough to gain clarity, but ADHD brains don't always work on that timeline. When your nervous system is highly dysregulated, it can take longer to reset, sometimes even days.

You may have heard the phrase "Don't let the sun go down on your anger." But for ADHD, that advice can backfire. Pushing for resolution while dysregulated can lead to over-explaining, misreading the situation, or making impulsive decisions. Sometimes, the best thing you can do is sleep on it, literally. Another night of rest can shift your perspective entirely because sleep helps reprocess emotions and regulate mood.

So, whether you need a day, a week, or just a good night's sleep, the goal is the same:

Regulate first, then respond.

Living in a constant state of stress isn't sustainable. It keeps your nervous system stuck in high gear, which can lead to emotional exhaustion, burnout, and eventual shutdown. Let's explore what happens next when your stress hits the wall.

ADHD in the Red Light

For most neurotypicals, red light looks like stopping completely. However, for ADHDers, it often looks like *functional freeze*, a state where your body keeps going, but your brain checks out.

You're still moving, working, and responding, but it's all mechanical, not intentional. To others, you seem fine, maybe even high functioning. But inside, you feel like a phone running on 1 percent battery with no charger in sight.

Even you might not recognize you're in shutdown. ADHD masking doesn't just hide hyperactivity; it also hides exhaustion, overwhelm, and emotional collapse. You might be pushing through out of habit until your body forces you to stop.

Functional Freeze

Many describe the red-light state as "a calm that surpasses all understanding." You're not panicked. You're not overwhelmed. You're just… *here.*

But there's a huge difference between ventral vagal calm (safety and connection), where you feel grounded, clear, and engaged, and dorsal vagal calm (shutdown and survival), where you feel detached, numb, and checked out:

- Ventral is like sitting by a campfire, relaxed and connected

- Dorsal is like watching a movie of your own life, barely present

Dorsal vagal calm is functional freeze. Your body is in autopilot survival mode, keeping you moving while your core functions are offline. If you're doing life, but it feels like muscle memory with no real awareness or presence, you may be experiencing functional freeze. Some other common signs include:

- **Cognitive shutdown.** Simple decisions feel impossible. Words won't come out. Your brain feels like it's buffering.

- **Emotional numbness**—not stressed, not excited—just empty. You're going through the motions.

- **Overwhelming sleepiness.** You feel like you took a heavy dose of sleeping pills out of nowhere.

- **ADHD paralysis.** Normally, your brain moves fast. But here? It's stuck in quicksand.

- **Task avoidance.** Bills, emails, calls…all ignored. You can't even think about them.

- **External referencing.** Instead of knowing what you need, you copy others. You say, "I don't care, you choose." Not because you're easygoing, but because decision-making is too much.

- **People-pleasing and fawning.** Saying no feels impossible. Boundaries feel unsafe. You over-focus on others' needs because you don't know your own.

- **Masking on overdrive.** You look "functional," maybe even productive. But it's all a front.

- **Memory blackouts and test anxiety.** Ever sat down for a test and forgotten everything? Or had a conversation and your brain went blank? That's your nervous system powering down under stress.

- **Yawning** (even when you're not tired). It's not rudeness, it's biofeedback. Your body is trying to stay engaged, not check out.

The Hidden Cost of Red

Since you *look* fine, no one realizes you're struggling, including you. You don't notice how drained you are because shutdown disguises itself as calm.

But functional freeze doesn't just disappear. Stress still lives in your body, piling up as:

- Chronic tension and pain

- Migraines

- Brain fog

- Energy crashes

- Skin and health issues

This isn't laziness or procrastination; it's a survival state.

TOOLBOX: Unfreezing

The first step out of freeze is recognizing it:

- ☑ **Ask yourself:** *Am I calm because I feel safe or because I've checked out?*

- ☑ **Reconnect with your body:** Notice your breath, stretch your fingers, take a sip of water and actually *taste* it.

- ☑ **Make one small choice** for yourself (even if it's just deciding between tea or coffee).

You don't have to fight your way out of freeze. You just must invite yourself back and anchor back to ventral.

ADHD Emotional Rollercoaster

If you feel like you swing between emotional extremes, you're not imagining it.

Your nervous system can't always transition smoothly between states, which means you might go from high-energy overwhelm to emotional shutdown in seconds (for example, a heated reaction one moment and total dissociation the next, or sudden exhaustion after emotional intensity). This cycle happens because the prefrontal cortex, the part of your brain that regulates emotions, is already working overtime (Shaw et al. 2014). When stress hits, your nervous system switches from intense reactivity to total collapse.

This constant tug-of-war between reaction and shutdown is why so many ADHDers struggle with self-regulation. It's not just about willpower or self-control. It's about having a nervous system that reacts before logic can catch up. When the overwhelm becomes too much, your system flips the switch from chaos to dorsal vagal shutdown.

Burnout

Your nervous system works like a volume knob. When you need energy to get things done, the volume turns up. You move into a high-energy, task-focused state. But if the volume stays too loud for too long, your system can crash. You might feel foggy, exhausted, or emotionally flat. That's burnout.

Burnout is not the same as being tired. It's when your body and brain go offline. You may:

- Sleep a lot but never feel rested

- Struggle to make decisions or finish basic tasks

- Avoid social interactions

- Feel emotionally numb or disconnected

- Lose interest in things you enjoy

- Constantly yawn

This can look similar to dorsal vagal shutdown, but there's a difference. Shutdown is a short-term response to feeling overwhelmed or unsafe. Burnout builds over time. It happens when your system runs on adrenaline for too long without enough recovery.

Because ADHDers often do not notice the cycle of yellow-light mode, crash, and struggling to recharge, burnout creeps up until it's too late.

People with ADHD often miss the signs. They power through, don't notice what their body is telling them, and hyperfocus on a sense of urgency until the crash hits. Learning to spot this pattern and recharge before burnout takes hold is essential for long-term regulation and well-being.

Learning to Regulate, Not Mask

Many ADHDers develop masking behaviors to cope, forcing themselves to be "on," copying others' behavior, or people-pleasing to avoid discomfort. But masking is a survival strategy, not connection.

The real key? Regulating your nervous system so that connection feels natural instead of forced. When you're in the green state, you don't have to think so hard about how to socialize—it just *happens*. You can listen without overanalyzing, speak without second-guessing, and leave interactions feeling energized rather than drained.

Understanding how your nervous system influences social interactions helps take the pressure off. Instead of assuming you "lack social skills," you can start recognizing when your nervous system is out of sync and use strategies to regulate rather than mask your way through it.

TOOLBOX: Energy Management

Instead of trying to pace yourself like a neurotypical, think about energy like a bank account:

- ☑ **Identify burnout warning signs.** If you start yawning, zoning out, or feeling disconnected, slow down before you crash.

☑ **Make deposits before you're broke.** Do not wait until exhaustion hits to rest. Build "green light" activities into your day before burnout sets in.

☑ **Use interest, not discipline.** Following motivation and interest keeps energy levels more stable. Pushing through tasks you hate drains energy faster.

☑ **Recovery takes time.** If you're burned out, you cannot "push through" recovery. You need more than one good night's sleep to reset.

Burnout and shutdown are signs that your nervous system needs care. You don't need to push harder—you need to come home to safety. That's what the green zone offers. But for us, the calm of green can feel disorienting. It may register more like shutdown than safety, simply because it's unfamiliar. Let's take a look at what actually happens when you're in the green zone.

ADHD Green Light

Calm isn't depression or laziness—it's just...calm. But when you're used to chaos, that quiet can feel unsettling. The green-light state (ventral vagal/social engagement) is where your nervous system is relaxed, present, and socially engaged. For most people, this feels ideal. But for ADHDers, it can feel foreign, even suspicious.

That go-go-go energy? On pause. The thrill-seeking drive? Gone. You might wonder if you're losing your edge. Friends and coworkers may even ask, "Are you okay?" And in your quieter state, you might second-guess yourself. *Is this burnout? Am I just being lazy?*

Green-Light Discomfort

The green-light state (ventral vagal/social engagement) is where your nervous system is calm, connected, and regulated. For most people, this is ideal. It's where focus, communication, and emotional stability thrive. But for ADHDers, it can feel foreign, unsettling, or even wrong.

Stillness Isn't Calm—It's Restless

For most people, stillness is soothing. It signals relaxation, safety, and ease. Slowing down thoughts calms them down. But for many ADHDers, stillness doesn't feel calming. It feels uncomfortable, even agitating. The moment we stop, our brain kicks into overdrive. Lying down to sleep? *Boom.* Suddenly, every thought we've ever had floods in. Trying to meditate? *Good luck!* Now we're replaying every awkward conversation from the past decade. Our minds don't settle just because we decide they should.

And the less external stimulation we have, the more our brain starts searching for it. High-energy interactions feel exciting, while calm conversations and slow moments can seem dull or even lonely. Without adrenaline, our brain might feel bored or restless, unconsciously looking for *something* to spark energy, even if that means creating stress. That's why stillness can feel like an itch that needs to be scratched.

So, when someone says "Just sit still and relax," they might as well be saying "Hold your breath and feel at peace." It just doesn't work that way.

Who Am I Without Stress?

If quick thinking, bold actions, and big energy have always defined you, the quiet of green light might leave you wondering *Am I still me?* Being in the green-light state might feel like losing part of yourself.

Fear of Stopping

Imagine an old car that needs a jump start to get going. Once it runs, it drives smoothly, but if it stops, it needs another jump. That is the ADHD brain. Getting started takes effort, but once in motion, it can accomplish amazing things. The challenge is that stopping feels risky because restarting is difficult.

Shifting into calm means losing the wave you're riding, the momentum that's driving you forward. You might worry that you'll forget what you were doing or struggle to pick it back up later. So, we push through, catching the wave and riding it hard, even if it looks manic to others.

For neurotypicals, stopping and starting tasks comes more easily; it's like their ocean is always calm and steady. But for us, the waves are unpredictable. When the surf's up, we have to ride it because we don't know when the next tide will come. This can make pacing ourselves feel impossible; our brains are built for sprints, not marathons.

No Pressure, No Action

If you've always relied on stress to get things done, calm can feel like hitting the brakes. Without urgency, motivation disappears.

Furthermore, calm feels like a threat: Your nervous system has learned that slowing down can lead to mistakes, forgotten tasks, or getting in trouble. Instead of feeling safe, green triggers alarms. *If we relax, we'll fall apart!*

Shutdown vs. Rest

When you finally step out of stress, your body may crash into exhaustion. But instead of recognizing this as *rest*, your brain may misinterpret it as failure or shutdown. It's easy to mix them up because both are part of the parasympathetic nervous system, and both involve a sense of calm or stillness. However, the key difference lies in the context: the green-light state emerges from safety, while the red-light state arises in response to danger or overwhelm.

Why Green Is Out of Reach

Polyvagal theory suggests that social connection and coregulation are the path to nervous system regulation. But for many ADHDers, the opposite may be true.

When you have social executive functioning impairments, interacting with others ramps up the pressure. Every moment becomes a performance—scanning for the right words, the right timing, the right tone. And in all that effort, the actual connection gets lost. It's like driving a stick shift in an unfamiliar car, through an unfamiliar city, during rush hour. You're hyperfocused on every move, constantly correcting and second-guessing. Instead of settling into the ride, your nervous system spikes into yellow or even red—and the last thing you're doing is enjoying the scenery.

That's why for many ADHDers, the green-light state—where you feel calm, connected, and socially engaged—can feel completely out of reach. Instead of syncing naturally with social flow, you feel overwhelmed, disconnected, and drained. Even positive interactions might not feel regulating because they come with performance demands your brain isn't equipped to meet on cue .

Neuroscience backs this up. Ventral vagal regulation—the foundation for social ease—is often impaired in neurodevelopmental conditions like ADHD (Porges 2011). That means your nervous system doesn't always grant you access to the calm and connection others feel automatically.

So how do you know your nervous system isn't in green, even if you're trying to connect?

Look for these signs:

- **Overcompensating:** You talk too much, overexplain, or force connection because silence feels threatening.

- **Withdrawing:** You zone out, get quiet, or feel like an outsider, even in a familiar group.

- **Fawning:** You over-accommodate or people-please to avoid disapproval or conflict.

These responses are clues that your system isn't feeling safe.

This also explains why many ADHDers find their green light in solitude. A walk alone, a quiet room, time with a pet—these feel safer than navigating unpredictable social terrain. That doesn't mean we can't connect. It just means we need to find *how* we connect. We need relationships that feel like *regulation*, not performance.

And sometimes, this is an area that needs healing. Social connection can become a green-light tool—but only with the right people. People who feel safe, who don't require masking, who give your nervous system permission to breathe. Finding those people, and learning to turn to them instead of away from them, is part of the work. That's how we begin to rewire what connection means—not as pressure, but as peace.

Conclusion

Your ADHD nervous system regulates energy, emotions, and social connection in a way that often feels out of sync with the world. If you've been using neurotypicals as a roadmap for how your brain should work, it's no wonder you've felt frustrated or confused. Your nervous system plays by different rules and neurotypical ventral anchors could be very different than yours. Give yourself permission to anchor differently. That's okay. The goal is to find what works for you and access your anchors when needed.

Learning how to identify your state and find your way back to safety helps you prevent burnout, regulate emotions before they spiral, and show up in relationships without having to mask who you are.

In the next chapter, we will dive into emotion regulation, why ADHD makes feelings so intense, how to navigate rejection sensitivity, and tools to help you stay grounded and connected even when your emotions are big.

Chapter 4

Emotion Management

With ADHD, emotions are front and center. You see them, feel them, and process them out loud. But once the moment passes, you might be hit with an emotional hangover—a flood of regret, vulnerability, and exhaustion that has you replaying conversations and questioning how you came across. You're left wondering if you overshared, overreacted, or came off wrong, wishing you could take it all back.

In moments like these, it's easy to blame emotions themselves. But emotions aren't the problem—the issue is what we do *with* them. Emotions are essential messengers. They fuel passion, creativity, and connection. They help us care, act, and respond. But without the skills to manage their intensity, they can overwhelm us and drive patterns like impulsiveness, avoidance, or deep self-doubt. Emotion regulation helps you adjust the volume so your emotions energize you without burning you—or others—out.

In this chapter, we'll dive into the biggest social-emotional challenges ADHDers face, including emotional triggers, rejection sensitive dysphoria (RSD), and shame activation. These emotional hot spots shape how we interact with others, often driving impulsive reactions, social anxiety, or self-criticism. With the right strategies, you can learn to navigate these moments so you can build emotional balance and resilience.

Emotions 101

Emotions are complex physiological responses that act as messengers, communicating information, motivating action, and guiding how we respond to our environment.

Emotions have three purposes:

- **Communication:** Emotions signal your internal state to others (e.g., sadness invites support and empathy).

- **Motivation:** Emotions drive adaptive behaviors (e.g., fear makes you flee danger, joy encourages connection).

- **Influence and control:** Emotional expression shapes situations (e.g., anger sets boundaries, sadness elicits comfort).

Emotions aren't good or bad; they simply carry information. How you respond to them determines their impact on your life.

> **Key takeaway:** *Feelings are not facts, and thoughts are not truths—they are information to attend to!*

Understanding emotions is the first step, but knowing what an emotion is doesn't automatically mean we know how to process, express, and respond to emotions in a balanced way.

About Emotion Regulation

Emotion regulation is the brain's ability to monitor, adjust, and manage emotions in a way that aligns with your goals and social expectations. ADHD can impair this function, leading to:

- Sudden emotional reactions (e.g., frustration or anger flaring up without warning)

- Difficulty self-soothing, making it hard to recover from emotional intensity

- Struggles shifting into more goal-aligned emotional states

Social emotion regulation is the ability to manage emotions within social interactions, including:

- Recognizing and understanding emotions (in yourself and others)

- Regulating emotional reactions during conversations and interactions

- Using emotional awareness to improve communication and relationships

Because the ADHD nervous system is dysregulated, social emotion management can feel especially challenging. Before diving into emotional dysregulation, let's cover the basics.

Processing and Releasing

Emotions carry energy that must be processed and released to complete their cycle, much like digestion:

- Ingestion (Activation) → Emotions arise from sensory input or triggering events

- Digestion (Processing) → The body and mind interpret and make sense of the emotion

- Excretion (Expression) → Emotional energy is released through expression

When this cycle isn't completed, emotions build up, causing what we might call "emotional constipation"—leaving you frozen, shut down, or numb. Or "emotional diarrhea"—spilling out uncontrollably. Suppressing feelings doesn't make them disappear; it traps them, leading to psychological distress or even physical symptoms. You move forward by actually feeling your emotions, sitting with them, understanding what they're trying to tell you, and then letting them move through and out of your system. That's what brings relief and resolution.

The operating principle here is that *what you resist persists!* Attempts to push away or suppress emotions could make them stronger and more overwhelming. Painful emotions are a natural part of life, but how you respond to them determines whether they become suffering. If you resist or fight against them, they tend to linger and intensify. Instead, acknowledging and allowing emotions to move through you can reduce their power and help you process them more effectively.

The Mind's Immune System

Emotional resilience is like your mind's immune system. Just like your body fights off illness, emotional resilience helps you stay emotionally regulated during tough times. When you're physically worn down—from poor sleep, stress, or poor nutrition—your body becomes more vulnerable to illness. The same goes for emotions: when resilience is low, frustration, anxiety, and anger are more likely to take hold.

Strong resilience is like strong immunity. It helps you stay grounded, tolerate distress, and bounce back when things aren't going well—knowing that, even when it feels overwhelming, you'll be okay.

Emotional resilience can be developed. By caring for your nervous system with rest, movement, good nutrition, and connection, you build emotional endurance. This makes it easier to stay steady, tolerate distress, and recover from setbacks with greater stability and less overwhelm. The bottom line: Taking care of your physical health is taking care of your emotional health.

Strong emotional resilience is like having strong immunity. It helps you face negative emotions, discomfort, and stress without losing your balance. You can stay grounded and even maintain a sense of humor, no matter what life throws at you.

Interrupted Development

The same factors you read about in chapter 3 that affect energy management (asynchronistic growth, neurological delays, and others) affect emotion regulation and social learning in similar ways. ADHD can impair social learning, and many ADHDers miss out on opportunities to develop mature emotional coping strategies. This can lead to reactive, impulsive responses rather than regulated, intentional emotional management.

One of the biggest challenges of interrupted emotional development is relying on external factors to navigate inner experiences, emotions, and needs. When emotion regulation wasn't modeled or supported in childhood, it can lead to an ongoing sense of dependency on others for stability, validation, and reassurance. ADHD can magnify this tendency, as struggles with self-regulation may make it harder to manage emotions internally.

When emotion development is interrupted, you might continue to approach your emotional needs and relationships with a mindset similar to what you had when you were younger. You might use the same approach to manage your emotions and needs. These strategies are often referred to as ingrained childhood survival strategies. You might find yourself:

- Unable to self-regulate emotions. Without the ability to self-soothe and self-regulate, you might feel hijacked by emotions, panicked when alone in your pain, and angry that others aren't there to help. Strong emotions take over quickly, leaving you feeling out of control, reactive, or emotionally exhausted.

- Requiring others to regulate your emotions. You might seek constant reassurance, validation, or soothing from others to feel okay.

- Struggling to express needs directly. You may expect others to "know" what you need without you having to state it clearly, leading to frustration and anger when they don't.

- Equating rejection with abandonment. Boundaries or unmet expectations can feel personal and devastating, triggering deep emotional pain disproportionate to the situation.

- Reacting rather than responding. Emotions feel immediate and urgent, making impulsive reactions more common than intentional, regulated responses.

When emotional development is interrupted, the past doesn't stay in the past—it shows up in the present, often in overwhelming or confusing ways. These intense reactions often reflect old emotional wounds reactivating in the present (what we will soon explore as emotional flashbacks). Understanding the link between ADHD and emotion regulation challenges can provide clarity, helping you to develop strategies to foster emotional resilience and self-regulation.

Triggers

Not all big emotions are caused by what's happening right now. Sometimes, a seemingly small moment can spark a wave of intensity that feels disproportionate or hard to explain. That's often because the moment activated a *trigger*—something your nervous system registered as a threat based on past experiences, not present danger.

For adults with ADHD, emotional triggers can be intense, fast, and confusing. They bypass logic and throw the nervous system into a survival state before the brain has time to make sense of what's happening. The result is often an emotional overreaction that feels overwhelming, out of place, or even a little embarrassing afterward.

In this section, we'll walk through four common types of emotional triggers that show up in everyday social interactions:

- Emotional flashbacks

- Hidden expectations and unenforceable rules

- RSD

- Digital dysregulation and social media

Each of these triggers can hijack your nervous system, distort perception, and make it harder to regulate emotions in the moment. But when you learn to spot them and understand what they're really about, you can start responding with clarity and self-leadership instead of reactivity.

Emotional Flashbacks

Emotional flashbacks occur when a present situation triggers overwhelming feelings tied to past experiences.

For example:

- A friend cancels plans, and instead of just feeling disappointed, you feel panic or rage, as if you've been abandoned.

- A partner asks for space, and it floods you with shame, rejection, or desperation.

- A delayed reply makes you feel invisible, discarded, or unworthy, even if that's not the intent.

These reactions feel out of proportion because they're triggered by old wounds, causing your body to relive intense emotions from the past. The emotion is real, but it's not about the present moment—it's your body reacting to something that once felt unsafe or overwhelming. Recognizing emotional flashbacks helps you step back and see that it's not the situation at hand, but an old wound being triggered. With this awareness, you can stop blaming yourself and understand what your nervous system needs to feel safe again.

The key to emotion regulation in tough moments is to recognize what's happening and reframe the experience, not to suppress feelings. When you feel abandoned, unseen, or panicked:

- ☑ **Pause and identify the emotional flashback.** *Is my reaction about this moment, or does it feel bigger than the situation?*

- ☑ **Ground yourself in the present.** *I'm no longer a powerless child. As an adult, I have choices and ways to meet my needs.*

Hidden Expectations and Unenforceable Rules

When emotions from childhood still drive adult experiences, they often shape rigid and unrealistic expectations about relationships, fairness, and validation. These beliefs, while understandable, can make emotion regulation harder and increase frustration, disappointment, and shame.

Here's how this plays out:

- *If they cared about me, they would just know what I need.* (Hidden expectation: Others should anticipate my emotions without me expressing them.)

- *If someone sets a boundary, it means I'm being rejected.* (Unenforceable rule: People must always be available to me, or else I'm unworthy.)

- *I should never feel lonely if I'm in a relationship.* (Hidden expectation: A romantic partner should fulfill all my emotional needs.)

- *If I do everything right, people will love and appreciate me.* (Unenforceable rule: Love and approval should be guaranteed if I meet expectations.)

These subconscious rules and expectations create emotional traps, leading to frustration when others don't behave according to the scripts we were conditioned to believe. When emotional development is interrupted, it's easy to get stuck in childhood-based emotional responses, expecting others to meet our needs in the way a caregiver once should have. But as adults, we're no longer helpless, powerless, or dependent on others for survival.

☑ **Challenge hidden expectations.** *Am I holding others to an unspoken rule they don't know about?*

☑ **Validate your emotions, but don't let them define reality.** *Feeling alone doesn't mean I'm abandoned. Feeling rejected doesn't mean I'm unworthy.*

Learning to recognize emotional flashbacks, challenge hidden expectations, and take ownership of our own regulation and needs allows us to break the cycle of emotional dependence and create relationships that are based on true connection, rather than old coping patterns of survival that no longer serve us. The goal is to stop childhood emotions from controlling our present.

Rejection Sensitive Dysphoria

Emotional dysregulation in ADHD is often heightened by RSD, where severe emotional pain is triggered by real or imagined rejection or criticism. RSD is an involuntary survival response that can manifest in everyday life as:

- Sudden waves of shame, rage, or sadness after rejection, even if minor

- Avoiding social situations to prevent the risk of rejection

- Obsessing over past interactions, replaying them in your mind

- Over-apologizing, people-pleasing, or perfectionism to prevent disapproval

Because RSD is rooted in the nervous system's response to perceived threats, whether real or imagined, it can distort reality. Let's explore how neuroception can make neutral situations feel like rejection or danger, further amplifying emotional dysregulation.

When your nervous system enters a yellow-light state (fight or flight), your brain shifts into threat-detection mode. This means neuroception starts distorting reality. When you feel threatened, your brain is no longer filtering information objectively; it's reacting for survival. When the brain perceives danger, it heightens certain sensory and social inputs while filtering out anything that contradicts the threat. This can make neutral situations feel hostile and amplify minor stressors into overwhelming experiences:

- **Sounds seem louder and harsher.** Your nervous system is primed for danger, making background noise unbearable. Even normal voices can sound like shouting.

- **Faces look angry or threatening.** Your brain scans for danger, misreading neutral or distracted expressions such as rejection, judgment, or hostility.

Your nervous system is doing its job. But your dysregulated brain needs a calm, regulated self to "take the wheel" before making decisions. Pull over. Regulate. And respond when the light turns green!

Digital Dysregulation and Social Media

For those with RSD, social media can feel like a constant referendum on their self-worth. A delayed response, an unanswered message, or a drop in engagement can feel like rejection, triggering intense emotional distress. But this reaction isn't just about thoughts, but also what your nervous system perceives as a threat.

Your neuroception relies on eye contact, vocal tone, body language, and even scent to determine whether you're safe. In real-life interactions, these cues are available naturally. But in digital communication like texts, emails, and social media, those cues are missing. Without them, your nervous system assumes something is off and sounds the alarm.

When your nervous system can't confirm safety, it doesn't stop, it doubles down. You might find yourself rereading texts to analyze tone, checking social media to see if someone is ignoring you, or scrolling endlessly, trying to find reassurance. Just like when you suspect someone might have farted, you start sniffing, your brain asking, *Did someone fart?* The same thing happens with social media—except the "sniffing" sounds like *Why haven't they responded yet? Why did they like their post but not mine?*

The more you check, the worse you feel, just like the more you sniff, the stronger the stink! The answer seems obvious: Pinch your nose and leave the room. But our instinct is to keep investigating, trying to make sense of things, even when that only makes it worse.

Instead of staying stuck in the scroll-check-analyze loop, try:

- ☑ **Noticing when you're spiraling.** The moment you catch yourself obsessing, pause.

- ☑ **Stepping away from the screen.** Even a short break can help reset your nervous system.

- ☑ **Seeking real human interaction.** A face-to-face conversation (even brief) provides the safety cues your nervous system is desperately looking for.

These moments can leave you feeling exposed and emotionally raw, especially when the nervous system can't find resolution. And when that emotional vulnerability collides with ADHD's tendency toward self-blame, it often opens the door to shame.

Shame

Shame can overwhelm in two ways: through shame attacks, which hit suddenly and intensely, or shame spirals, which are slow and insidious. A shame attack feels like an emotional panic attack, gripping you in the moment. A shame spiral lingers, pulling you into deeper self-condemnation over time.

Shame Attacks

A *shame attack* is a sudden wave of intense shame, often triggered by a social misstep, mistake, or perceived rejection. It hijacks your thoughts, body, and behavior, making it difficult to shake off. While everyone experiences shame differently, there are some common ways it tends to show up:

- **Thoughts:** obsessing over the event, fearing rejection, or catastrophizing ("this ruined everything")

- **Body:** dorsal vagal shutdown (withdrawal, numbness), brain fog, nausea, or sleep disturbances

- **Behavior:** isolating, avoiding responsibilities, impulsively apologizing or over-explaining, or projecting shame outward as anger or blame

Shame attacks can last for days or weeks. If left unchecked, they may harden into core beliefs of being unworthy, leading to a shame spiral.

Shame Spirals

Unlike a shame attack's sudden flood, a *shame spiral* slowly reinforces negative self-beliefs, keeping you stuck in a cycle of self-criticism and avoidance. You might notice them as:

- **Thoughts:** ruminating over a lifetime of mistakes, chronic self-judgment, believing you're "fundamentally broken"

- **Emotions:** feeling unworthy, socially anxious, or emotionally numb

- **Behavior:** avoiding relationships, sabotaging opportunities, perfectionism, or people-pleasing to prevent criticism

A shame spiral doesn't just hijack your emotions, it erodes your self-worth over time. Recognizing these patterns is the first step toward breaking free.

Growing Emotional Maturity

Emotional maturity isn't about controlling emotions, being perfect, or never needing help. It's about learning how to notice, regulate, and respond to emotions with care and intention rather than being ruled by them.

If you ever wonder, *Where is the adult in this situation?* turn your attention inward. You're now the adult. And that means you're the one who can step in, reassure yourself, and take the necessary steps to meet your own needs.

Your inner child may still be waiting for someone else to show up, to soothe the fear, to validate the pain, to make things right. But now, you're here. And you can let them know, "You're not alone anymore. I see you. I hear you. I will take care of what you need."

This shift from seeking external rescue to self-leadership is what true emotional maturity looks like. It doesn't mean doing everything alone or rejecting connection, but it does mean turning toward yourself first, like a loving parent tending to their child.

Nurturing Your Emotions

Imagine a child crying because they scraped their knee. A harsh parent might say, "Stop crying! You're fine!" while a loving parent would kneel down, acknowledge their pain, and offer comfort: "I know that hurts, and it makes sense you're upset. Let's take care of it together."

Now imagine this with your own emotions. When you speak to yourself with patience and care rather than judgment and dismissal, you're reparenting yourself in real time. Here are some tips on how to nurture emotions:

- ☑ **Attend to your needs with care.** Just as a good parent wouldn't leave their child to struggle alone, you can show up for yourself—whether that means self-soothing, setting boundaries, or seeking healthy support.

- ☑ **Notice what you feel** instead of ignoring, suppressing, or becoming overwhelmed by it. Imagine a loving parent noticing their child's distress: "You're upset! Are you okay?"

- ☑ **Label emotions accurately** so you can respond appropriately rather than catastrophizing or shutting down: "You're not bad—I see that you're just frustrated and sad. Let's figure this out."

☑ **Regulate emotions effectively** so they don't hijack your decisions, relationships, or sense of self (see the Emotion Regulation Toolbox in the next section). Self-soothing is like holding your own hand through discomfort rather than expecting someone else to fix it.

You're not changing the past—you're changing the future by stepping into the role of the adult you needed.

TOOLBOX: Emotion Regulation Skills

Below are key approaches on how to regulate emotions, grouped into different categories to help you apply the right tools when needed.

Building Emotional Resilience

These strategies strengthen your nervous system, making emotional ups and downs easier to manage:

☑ **Ventral vagal exercises**—practices like deep breathing, yoga, and cold exposure to build emotional resilience

☑ **Healthy lifestyle habits**—sleep, nutrition, hydration, and movement for emotional stability

☑ **Daily emotional check-ins**—journaling or body scanning to increase self-awareness and prevent emotional buildup

☑ **Joy and play**—engaging in fun, creative activities (music, movement, humor) to promote nervous system balance

☑ **Self-compassion and affirmations**—shifting from self-criticism to supportive inner dialogue

☑ **Education and awareness**—learning about your nervous system and emotional patterns to improve self-regulation

Body-Based Regulation

When emotions hit hard, these techniques help shift your emotional reactivity and your physiological state in the moment:

☑ **Self-soothing techniques**—grounding, rhythmic movement, deep-pressure touch

☑ **Change-the-state interventions**—ice on the face, sucking something sour, paced breathing

☑ **Vagus nerve hacks** (vagal tone exercise)—gargling, humming, or chanting to quickly regulate the nervous system

☑ **Anchoring techniques**—holding a smooth rock, bracelet, or grounding scent for sensory regulation

Thought Interventions

Your thoughts shape your emotions. When they're influenced by assumptions or self-blame, emotions can spiral. These practices can help shift unhelpful thinking patterns and reduce distress:

☑ **Reframe your thinking**—catch automatic negative thoughts and replace them with balanced ones

☑ **Use grounding scripts**—try phrases like "This is uncomfortable, but I can handle it"

☑ **Spot hidden expectations**—notice rules like "They should know how I feel," which often lead to frustration

☑ **Check the facts**—ask if your thoughts align with reality

☑ **Take opposite action**—do the opposite of what your impulse suggests to regain control

Let's dive deeper into the last two tools:

Check the facts. Feelings are real but not always true. Here's how to slow down and get clear:

- *What am I feeling?*

- *What just happened?*

- *What story is my brain telling?*

- *What else could explain it?*

Example: Someone looks at their phone during your presentation.

- Thought: *They're bored. I blew it.*

- Fact check: *I don't know why they looked.*

- Reframe: *Maybe it was urgent—it might not be about me.*

Take opposite action

Sometimes emotions urge you to hide, avoid, or lash out. If the feeling doesn't match the facts, do the opposite:

- Shame says hide → Reach out

- Fear says avoid → Take a step toward

- Anger says lash out → Pause and soften

Acting from your values, not your emotions, builds emotional strength.

Relationship-Based Regulation (Coregulation and Social Support)

Emotion regulation doesn't always happen alone—healthy connection plays a big role:

☑ **Coregulation with safe people**—seeking comfort from trusted individuals to restore balance

☑ **Seeking validation without dependence**—learning to accept support while strengthening self-regulation

☑ **Boundary awareness**—recognizing when to lean on others versus when to self-soothe

Conclusion

Understanding your emotions is key to managing them effectively. Some of the tools you've learned in this chapter build long-term resilience, while others provide immediate relief or help shift ingrained patterns. The more you practice, the more flexible and adaptable your nervous system becomes.

These strategies are just a starting point. For more detailed exercises and resources, visit http://www.newharbinger.com/56166. You can also revisit core skill #3 from chapter 1 for more practice with self-compassion.

You are not stuck. By learning to become your own emotion coach, relationships will no longer feel like a test of your worth but a space for giving and receiving without fear.

Shifting from reactivity to responsiveness takes practice. It means strengthening your nervous system through ventral vagal exercises and developing emotional maturity over time. As you build awareness and learn to recognize, name, and process your emotions, they stop feeling like enemies or absolute truths. They become messengers. And you become the one who listens, leads, and responds wisely.

You can learn to feel to heal, name it to tame it, co-regulate to regulate, and shift it to lift it. The goal isn't to silence your emotions—it's to move with them. To hold space for both the messy and the meaningful, trusting that no matter what shows up, you've got this.

Chapter 5

Response Inhibition

We've all seen it in real life or on TV—the easy, effortless friendships where people gather, swap stories, and genuinely connect. Whether at a favorite coffee shop, during game nights, or in those late-night conversations that stretch until morning, these moments capture the kind of social connection many long for. But for some, building that kind of bond feels just out of reach, even though they want it deeply.

Imagine someone who's trying everything to fit in. They might think, *If I'm funny, if I tell interesting stories, or if I relate to others' experiences, I'll be accepted.* They try to connect by sharing their thoughts and excitement, but something keeps going wrong. Instead of being seen as engaging, they're told they're dominating the conversation, or they come off as intimidating. What they thought would create connection only created distance.

Sound familiar?

For this person, their brain is like a runaway freight train powered by rapid-fire thoughts and an uncontrollable urge to share. Once an idea pops up, it feels impossible to hold it back. Paired with the tendency to jump between exciting thoughts, the conversation is pure chaos. Every comment someone makes triggers an immediate connection in their mind: "That reminds me of this incredible experience!" or "I know exactly what you mean!"

Inhibition, or the brain's "social filter," is the skill that helps your brain pause and resist impulses. But when you pair an ADHD brain bursting with excitement and ideas with poor inhibition, it's like the brakes are out. Before you know it, the words fly out faster than you can catch them. Your enthusiasm is genuine, but without a strong filter, it unintentionally steamrolls the conversation.

The good news is that inhibition skills can be trained. With intentional practice, we can strengthen our brain's ability to pause and respond thoughtfully.

In this chapter, we'll explore the hidden driver behind these challenges. We'll uncover how ADHD impacts our brain's "pause button" and how we can practice skills to strengthen response inhibition. At the end of the chapter, you'll have practical tools to navigate social interactions with intention, without dimming your light or losing your authenticity. You can also find a quick guide to inhibition on the website, http://www.newharbinger.com/56166.

Pause Button

In social settings, inhibition is critical. It's the executive function skill that helps you hold back impulses, filter your responses, and keep interactions flowing smoothly. Whether it's resisting the urge to interrupt, curbing oversharing, or pausing before reacting emotionally, social inhibition is what allows you to align your behavior with social expectations and build stronger connections.

Inhibition is like a mental brake pedal, giving your brain the split-second pause needed to stop, think, and choose your actions intentionally. In addition to halting physical impulses like interrupting or fidgeting, inhibition also helps manage internal distractions and emotional reactions.

Here's how it works:

- *Thought inhibition* filters out mental noise—thoughts such as *I should Google this!* or *Did I send that email?*—so you can stay focused.

- *Emotional inhibition* creates space to pause before reacting to feelings like anger or excitement, preventing impulsive actions you might regret.

- *Behavioral inhibition* helps you resist physical urges, like checking your phone during a meeting or blurting out a thought mid-conversation.

Without strong inhibition, life can feel chaotic. You might interrupt mid-sentence, chase rabbit holes of thoughts that derail your focus, or react emotionally in ways you later regret. Others might misunderstand these behaviors, seeing them as selfish, inattentive, or overly emotional. In reality, they're symptoms of a brain working overtime to process stimuli and struggling to prioritize what's most important.

Inhibition vs. Emotion Regulation

Inhibition and emotion regulation are closely related but distinct executive functions. Inhibition focuses on controlling *what you do*, while emotion regulation centers on *how you feel* and respond emotionally. Think of it this way:

- Inhibition—helps you pause and stop behaviors or reactions before they happen

- Emotion regulation—guides how you manage and process emotions once they arise

For example, inhibition might stop you from blurting out a sarcastic comment in a tense moment, while emotion regulation helps you process the frustration that triggered the impulse. Both work together: inhibition gives you pause, and emotion regulation steers your emotional response in a constructive direction.

The Three Components of Inhibition

At its core, inhibition involves three key skills that help you navigate interactions with intention and thoughtfulness:

- **Impulse regulation:** stopping immediate reactions. Impulse regulation is the ability to hit pause on that knee-jerk response, whether or not it's socially appropriate. It helps with timing and keeping the conversation on track.

  Example: You're in a meeting, and someone says something you strongly disagree with. Your first instinct is to jump in and set them straight, but impulse regulation helps you take a breath and think: *Is now the right time to speak, or should I wait until they finish?*

- **Response inhibition:** filtering out socially inappropriate responses. This skill helps you avoid saying or doing things that might violate social norms or make others uncomfortable. Take a second to think: *Is this the right thing to say in this context?*

  Example: You're chatting with someone you just met, and suddenly you're about to launch into a deeply personal story about your worst breakup. But before you do, you realize: *It's probably not the best time for this.* Social response inhibition lets you switch gears and steer the conversation toward something lighter. Crisis averted!

- **Self-restraint:** keeping your cool in emotionally charged moments. Self-restraint is what keeps you calm and collected when emotions are running high, preventing impulsive actions that could escalate the situation.

  Example: A friend makes a sarcastic comment that hits a nerve. Your instinct might be to snap back, but self-restraint gives you that moment to pause, take a deep breath, and respond calmly instead. Conflict is avoided, and friendship is preserved.

Together, these three skills help you stay in control, handle social situations thoughtfully, and build stronger connections. Each one plays a specific role in keeping your interactions respectful, smooth, and aligned with your goals.

Retraining Your Brains

I used to love curling up by the fireplace and getting lost in a good book. But somewhere along the way, my brain began to prefer the quick hits of social media reels and endless feeds. I know I'm not alone; so many of us have felt this shift. But what caused this change?

The way we consume information has evolved dramatically, moving from slower, deliberate formats to fast-paced, bite-sized content. Just as adding sugar to food keeps people coming back for more, fast-paced media stimulates the brain's dopamine system, making it harder to engage with slower formats. Social media and short-form content deliver news and entertainment in quick, dopamine-packed bursts. These bursts train our brains to crave more novelty and stimulation, making it harder to focus on slower content like books or long articles (Nikkelen et al. 2014). Over time, this cycle rewires how we think and leaves us constantly chasing the next hit of dopamine.

For ADHD brains, this is an especially sticky trap. With our naturally low dopamine levels and craving for stimulation, the "short burst" way of processing information is like a magnet. The more we feed it, the stronger it gets. That reinforcement makes it even harder to slow down, pause, and hold back in real-time moments.

The good news is our brain can relearn how to slow down, focus, resist distractions, and strengthen impulse control. Thanks to neuroplasticity, the brain's ability to reorganize and create new pathways, we can literally train ourselves to put on the brakes more easily.

Think of it like learning to ride a bike. At first, you wobble. It's awkward and hard. Your brain has to fire up all kinds of circuits for balance, movement, and coordination. Every pedal, every turn takes conscious effort. But with practice, those neural pathways strengthen. The neurons involved in steering, balancing, and pedaling begin to fire together more efficiently. Eventually, the process becomes automatic. You don't have to think about riding; your body just knows what to do.

Inhibition works the same way. Every time you practice hitting pause, whether it's holding back a comment, resisting a distraction, or taking a breath instead of reacting, you strengthen the pathways in your brain that support self-regulation. Over time, it becomes easier for your brain to "put on the brakes" when it counts.

Here's how it plays out:

- **Starting out:** Resisting impulses feels uncomfortable and difficult. Your brain's inhibition circuits are still under construction.

- **Keep practicing:** Each time you pause or resist an urge, those circuits get stronger. The more they fire together, the faster and easier they work.

- **Automatic response:** Eventually, pausing becomes second nature. The impulse is still there, but your brain now knows how to slow it down.

Practice also gives you a chance to prepare strategies in advance for those moments when impulsiveness shows up uninvited. When you know your common triggers and have a few go-to tools ready, it's much easier to stay grounded and connected.

You're not silencing yourself, rather, you're channeling your brilliance in a way that leaves room for others to shine too. And like any skill, your brain's pause power gets stronger with practice. Let's walk through a few ways to build it without dimming your light.

Practicing Impulse Regulation

One of the first times I focused on practicing impulse regulation was during a gathering with friends. My goal was simple: actively listen without chiming in at every opportunity. I literally had to force myself to sit there, sip my coffee, and stay quiet. It wasn't easy; my ADHD brain was buzzing with ideas, connections, and stories I wanted to share. The urge to jump in felt almost unbearable.

But I reminded myself why I was practicing: to connect more meaningfully with others, show that I valued their contributions, and avoid overwhelming them with my unrestrained excitement. I reassured myself that this was just practice. *This time*, I told myself, *I'll stay quiet. Next time, I'll find the right moment to share.* Over time, these practices paid off.

Meditation

A lot of people say, "I can't meditate! My mind just won't quiet down." But that's actually the point. The goal of meditation isn't to have no thoughts; instead, it's to notice where your mind goes and gently guide it back. With practice, this redirection becomes easier, and your attention grows stronger.

For ADHD brains, meditation is especially valuable. It trains you to observe distractions without reacting impulsively, helping to improve focus, impulse control, and mental clarity. Even a few minutes a day can build the neural pathways necessary for better self-regulation. Here are some tips to get started:

- ☑ **Start small:** Begin with one to five minutes daily and increase gradually.

- ☑ **Be consistent:** Regular practice matters more than duration.

- ☑ **Set realistic goals:** Progress may be slow, but small improvements add up.

- ☑ **Track progress:** Use a habit tracker or journal to stay motivated.

Over time, meditation shifts from feeling like a chore to becoming a rewarding part of your routine.

Tolerance for Silence

Silence can feel awkward—like showing up underdressed or wearing soggy socks. But learning to stay present in quiet moments is a powerful way to strengthen your pause muscle. Practice by holding back in conversations just a little longer than feels comfortable. Try being the last to speak in a group, or count to five before responding. The more you do it, the less awkward it feels—and the more grounded you'll become.

Watch a Movie Start to Finish (No Multitasking)

Choose a movie, set your phone aside, and resist the urge to multitask. No folding laundry, no scrolling, no checking email. Just watch. It sounds simple, but for ADHD brains, it's real training in presence. Make it to the credits and give yourself a little high five—you just gave your brain a full session of focus reps.

Let Others Go First

In group conversations, challenge yourself to hang back and really listen before jumping in. Not because your thoughts don't matter, but because practicing the pause helps you choose your moment with more impact. Think of it like timing a punchline—waiting a beat can make all the difference.

These mini-challenges may seem small, but they add up. Each one helps your brain build response inhibition and makes it easier to slow down when it matters. Over time, you'll find that pausing doesn't dampen your spark—it helps it land.

Effective Listening

Effective listening means more than just hearing words; it means being fully present in the conversation. One of the biggest challenges is resisting the urge to jump in with thoughts, stories, or solutions before the other person has finished speaking. Practicing response inhibition helps you slow down, engage more meaningfully, and create space for deeper connections.

Try this active listening challenge the next time you're in a conversation:

☑ **Listen without mentally rehearsing.** Instead of planning your response while the other person is talking, focus on absorbing their words. If you catch yourself forming a reply, gently redirect your attention back to them.

☑ **Repeat their main point internally.** As they speak, silently summarize their key point in your head. For example, if they say, "I had the hardest time at work today because my boss changed a deadline last minute," mentally note, *Boss changed deadline—stressful day.*

☑ **Use a nonverbal cue before speaking.** When they finish talking, pause before responding. Take a breath or nod. This brief pause strengthens response inhibition and signals that you're fully engaged.

☑ **Respond with a follow-up question.** Instead of immediately sharing a personal story or opinion, ask something that encourages them to continue:

- "That sounds frustrating. How did you handle it?"
- "That's a lot to deal with. What happened next?"
- "Wow, that's a big shift. How do you feel about it now?"

Practicing these shifts in how you listen and respond helps you slow down the moment and stay present in it. Now let's look at how to do the same when emotions get loud and reactions feel urgent.

Practicing Self-Restraint

Self-restraint is the skill that helps you regulate your emotional response before you speak or act. Where impulse regulation stops you from blurting something out, self-restraint helps you stay calm long enough to choose a response that aligns with your values and goals. It's the emotional pause that lets you steer the conversation in a constructive direction.

One way to practice this is through the "pause-reflect-respond" method, which helps you shift from reactive to intentional communication:

1. **Pause.** Take a deep breath, sip water, or count to 5. This interrupts the impulse and gives you a moment to regulate.

2. **Reflect.** Ask yourself:

    *   *What's my goal in this conversation?*

    *   *Is this response helpful, or am I reacting emotionally?*

    *   *Would I say this the same way if I had time to think?*

3. **Respond.** Choose your words based on what best serves the situation. If needed, reframe your response before speaking.

Here's an example of what this might look like.

Impulsive reaction:

Coworker: That project deadline is moving up.

You: Are you kidding me? That's completely unfair!

Self-restrained response:

Coworker: That project deadline is moving up.

You: (pausing, reflecting, regulating emotions, and responding thoughtfully) That's a big shift. What's our next step to adjust for it?

To go a little deeper with this method, try these tips:

☑ Before responding, **ask yourself one filtering question**: *Am I responding in a way that aligns with my goals and values?*

☑ If you feel emotionally charged, **write down your response first** before speaking or sending a message.

☑ In group discussions, **challenge yourself to wait** until at least two people have spoken before jumping in.

Over time, practicing self-restraint in conversations will help you shift from reactive to intentional, socially effective communication. It's about choosing responses that strengthen relationships rather than escalating conflicts.

Conclusion

Improving response inhibition is absolutely possible. With intention and practice, you can train your brain to pause, choose, and respond in ways that reflect your values, not just your impulses.

Every time you stop yourself from interrupting, resist the urge to overshare, or take a breath before reacting emotionally, you're reinforcing the neural pathways that support social success. You're building a brain that pauses before it speaks. And that pause makes all the difference.

This isn't about silencing your personality. It's about learning to express yourself in a way that creates space for others, builds trust, and makes conversations feel like connection not collision.

It won't be perfect. There'll be slipups, awkward moments, and days when your filter is on vacation. That's okay. Progress is in the practice. With every pause, you're rewiring for presence, connection, and thoughtful communication.

Chapter 6

Working Memory

You're in the middle of a conversation, fully engaged. Then—*poof!*—your brain skips over what was just said. You nod along, hoping context clues will save you. Or maybe someone is talking, and you're desperately holding onto a thought because if you don't say it *right now*, it will evaporate forever. So, you interrupt. *Again.*

It's frustrating, unpredictable, and not something you're doing on purpose.

This is the world of social working memory struggles, where everyday conversations turn into high-stakes mental gymnastics.

The problem is, this system is fragile. It's easily overloaded, distracted, or completely offline when you need it most. It's like having too many tabs open on your mental browser—someone's talking, another tab pops up with a memory or reminder, and just as you're about to respond, your system crashes.

In this chapter, we're going to unpack what's really going on with your social working memory. You'll learn:

- How ADHD affects your ability to track conversations in real time

- Why your brain struggles in certain social situations (and that it's not your fault)

- Practical tools to make interactions feel less overwhelming and more manageable

We'll walk through five core areas where social working memory tends to break down and give you strategies to make social life feel a little easier, one conversation at a time.

Mental Notepad

Working memory is your brain's temporary storage system. It helps you hold and process information in real time—whether you're trying to follow a conversation, remember what you were just doing, complete a multi-step task, or figure out what you were about to say.

Think of it as a mental notepad. It lets you jot down thoughts just long enough to use them. Unlike long-term memory, which stores things for later, working memory is all about the *now*. It's what keeps you on track as you speak, write, listen, and respond in the moment.

But that notepad has limited space and fills up fast.

Now imagine it's also your brain's mental computer, with each thought or task as an open browser tab. A few tabs? No problem. But when you're tracking a conversation, planning your response, filtering distractions, and remembering your point—all at once—your system slows down or crashes. ADHD makes this system even more sensitive.

Let's say you're watching YouTube and find a video you want to return to later. A few videos later, it's gone, and you can't remember what it was or how you found it. Luckily, YouTube has a history tab. Your brain doesn't. Without external support, that info just vanishes. That's what working memory failure feels like.

The challenge is that working memory has a strict capacity limit. Miller's Law suggests we can juggle about five to nine pieces of information before details start dropping (Miller 1956). That's why phone numbers are seven digits, and why you can remember your grocery list until someone asks for your zip code and suddenly it's all gone.

Social working memory helps keep conversations flowing. It tracks names, remembers past discussions, keeps you on topic, and manages what you say in real time. Ideally, it lets you engage smoothly in social interactions without forgetting key details or blurt out a thought before it disappears. And sometimes...it does.

Now let's look at some behind-the-scenes factors that make working memory challenging for ADHD brains. These include things like processing speed, attentional blinks, cognitive load, and cognitive intrusions. Each of these can interfere with how quickly you take in information, how well you understand it, and how much your brain can hold onto in the moment, especially during conversations.

Processing Speed

Processing speed refers to how quickly your brain takes in, organizes, and responds to information. Ever laughed at a joke a full minute after everyone else? It's not that you didn't get it, it just took a little longer for the joke to travel from hearing to understanding. That's a processing lag. Your brain received the information; it just needed more time to make sense of it, but for some, it takes longer for their comprehension to retrieve information.

If you have *auditory processing* challenges—or a condition called auditory processing disorder (APD)—this lag can be even more frustrating. APD means the brain has trouble decoding sounds, especially spoken words, even when hearing is perfectly normal. It makes it harder to retain spoken details, especially when there's background noise.

In noisy environments or fast-paced conversations, this can feel like trying to see words through a fog. You're listening, but it's like the message arrives scrambled or incomplete, and your brain has to work overtime just to make sense of it.

Reasons processing speed may lag include:

- Your brain is still unpacking one part of the conversation while the discussion has already moved on.

- Auditory processing challenges make it harder to retain spoken details, especially when there's background noise.

- It's like your brain is opening too many tabs at once—when that happens, it gets harder to keep track of what's being said or respond quickly.

Lagging processing speed may show up for you like this:

- By the time you're ready to respond, the topic has already changed.

- You miss key details because your brain is still processing the last thing that was said.

- You think of the perfect response—ten minutes too late.

TOOLBOX: Strategies for Processing Speed

- ☑ **Take a processing pause.** Instead of rushing, say "Let me think for a second" or "Hold on, I'm catching up."

- ☑ **Use active listening tricks.** Repeat key phrases in your head to stay engaged. *They're talking about their trip to Italy...*

- ☑ **Ask for a quick recap.** If you missed something, say "Can you repeat that last part?"

- ☑ **Follow up later.** If you think of something great after the fact, send a quick text: "Hey, I was thinking more about what we talked about..." Most people appreciate this.

Attentional Blinks

Sometimes, your brain is fully tuned in, and you're paying attention, but you still miss what comes next. An *attentional blink* is a split-second gap in awareness that happens right after you register something important. While your brain is still processing that first detail, it temporarily shuts out the next. You don't mean to miss it—you just literally didn't see or hear it.

Daniel Goleman and Richard Davidson (2017) explain this with the classic "Where's Waldo?" game. Imagine you're scanning a chaotic picture and—boom!—you spot Waldo. Your brain celebrates, but in that moment of "Yes! I found him," your attention blinks. You pause just long enough to miss another Waldo sitting right next to him.

Real life works the same way. Someone says, "My name is Jenny and I work in neurology," and you register "Jenny"…but not the rest. Your brain was still celebrating catching the name and missed the job title.

Research suggests people with ADHD experience more attentional blinks than those without (Goleman and Davidson 2017). ADHD brains tend to lock onto one detail and unintentionally block out the rest. This may look like distractibility, but it's actually over-focus.

TOOLBOX: Counteracting Attentional Blinks

So, what can you do about attentional blinks? So what helps? One effective method is practicing *open monitoring*—training your brain to stay alert without locking in too hard.

You can try:

☑ **A short body-and-breath reset.** In one study, people sat quietly for seventeen minutes, focused on their breath or body sensations (like their feet on the floor), and gently returned attention when it wandered. After just one session, they had fewer attentional blinks.

☑ **Softening your focus.** Instead of zooming in, practice a panoramic view. Look straight ahead and notice what's at the edges of your vision—*without moving your eyes.*

To try it, pick a spot in front of you and keep your gaze still. Then, without shifting your eyes, see if you can notice what's happening at the edges of your vision: the floor, the ceiling, your peripheral surroundings.

This widened awareness tells your brain that you're safe, reduces hyperfocus, and helps you stay tuned in during conversations—so you're less likely to miss what comes next.

Cognitive Load

Cognitive load is the mental effort required to juggle multiple details at once. Imagine carrying a heavy stack of books; at some point, your arms give out and things start dropping. The brain works the same way. When too much information floods in at once, working memory may not have the strength to hold the weight of too many details.

When cognitive load becomes overwhelming, your nervous system reacts:

- The yellow-light state kicks in, ramping up energy to keep up.

- If the strain continues, the red-light state takes over, leading to zoning out or shutting down. This isn't a choice—it's your brain protecting itself from overload.

Cognitive Intrusion

Cognitive intrusions are those random, unrelated thoughts that hijack your attention and pull you out of the moment. While you're trying to stay focused, your brain is busy making connections behind the scenes. Someone mentions a vacation, and suddenly you're remembering a meal you had in Thailand, which leads to thinking about what to cook for dinner. Five minutes later, you realize you've completely missed the conversation—and now you're panicking, trying to catch up or cover for what you didn't hear.

As you can see, working memory plays a big role in tracking conversations. Things like slower processing speed, cognitive overload, auditory challenges, and intrusive thoughts can seriously interfere with how it functions. These hidden factors can make social interactions feel mentally exhausting even when you're trying your best. Now that we've looked at what interferes with working memory, let's dig into the real-life challenges this creates in social situations.

Social Working Memory Challenges

Now, we'll walk through five common ways social working memory tends to break down, like mixing up words, going off topic, or forgetting people's names, and how these patterns show up for ADHD brains. Each one includes tools and strategies to help you navigate conversations with more ease and less stress.

Verbal Mismatch and Cross-Wiring

One of my most embarrassing moments happened at a sushi restaurant. My friends ordered octopus, and when it arrived, I blurted out, "Eww! How can you eat those testicles?" The whole room erupted in laughter, and even the sushi chefs joined in, gleefully shouting, "Testicles!" I had no idea what I'd said wrong until my friend leaned over and whispered, "It's tentacles, not testicles." Of course, I knew that. But in that moment, my brain grabbed the wrong word.

When your brain processes information quickly, it sometimes grabs the wrong word—often one that sounds similar or belongs in the same category. Your brain knows the right word, but somewhere between thought and speech, things get scrambled. These verbal mix-ups can be funny, frustrating, or painfully embarrassing, especially when they lead others to think you're not paying attention or aren't intelligent. You might laugh along, but it stings.

All brains group words by meaning or sound (Huth et al. 2016), but ADHD brains rely even more on these associations. Think of words as living in "neighborhoods." If you're looking for the word "cup," your brain might accidentally grab "bowl"—a close neighbor, but not quite right.

On top of that, the human brain tends to prioritize speed over accuracy, a phenomenon known as the *speed-accuracy trade-off*. This concept explains how your brain balances doing things quickly and doing them correctly. Research indicates that when we move or make faster decisions, we're more likely to make mistakes due to built-in processing limits and neural noise (Guiard and Rioul 2015). In other words, the faster we go, the more errors we make. If we slow down to be more accurate, tasks take more time.

Then there are those other times (hello, dysregulated brain) when everything slows to a crawl—and *word retrieval* flat-out refuses to cooperate. You know the word. It's right there. But your brain won't hand it over. It's like a shy cat hiding under the couch: the more you try to coax it out, the deeper it retreats.

It's right on the tip of my tongue…I swear it starts with an S.

Five hours later: *Spatula! That's the word.*

It's not that you didn't know the word; your brain just couldn't access it fast enough.

☑ **Try using descriptive workarounds** ("the thing you use to flip pancakes").

☑ And if it doesn't come? **Let it go.** It'll show up—probably in the shower.

Another version of this verbal mix-up is the *malaphor*—when your brain mashes two idioms into one confused (and often hilarious) phrase, like:

- "Let's burn that bridge when we get to it" (a blend of "Let's cross that bridge when we get to it" and "burning bridges"), or

- "It's not rocket surgery" (a mix of "It's not rocket science" and "It's not brain surgery")

These creative hybrids happen when your brain tries to pull up a familiar phrase but grabs parts of two instead. Honestly, some of them should be real. "Burn that bridge when we get to it"? Kinda poetic. When this happens:

☑ **Laugh it off.** Most people do.

☑ **Clarify if needed:** "Oops, I mashed up two sayings—meant to say [correct one]."

These slipups happen more often when working memory is overloaded or when your brain is trying to move fast and skips the double-check step. The brain often fills in the blanks with its best guess, like your phone's autocorrect, but without an undo button. And when your mental tabs are maxed out, holding onto the right word long enough to say it correctly becomes even harder. ADHD brains are especially prone to this because we retrieve words by association, think out loud, and sometimes prioritize speed over accuracy (Alt 2009; Pritchard et. al 2012).

Now let's shift from word mix-ups to another challenge—processing thoughts in real time. For many of us, speaking isn't the result of thinking, it is the thinking.

Externalized Processing

Some people think first, then speak. Others speak to think—their words act like breadcrumbs leading them to their point. This is called *external verbal processing*, where talking is thinking. Because ADHD brains struggle to filter and hold onto thoughts, it often feels like everything has to come out at once or we'll forget something important.

Many of us also rely on *narrative thinking*, meaning we process information as a story. We need to start at the beginning and work our way through to stay organized. Jumping into the middle feels impossible, and leaving out context makes everything feel disjointed. Add an interruption, and it's like someone erased our mental whiteboard—we have to start over so we can track what we are saying with a beginning, middle, and end. This often frustrates others—*What's your point!* We are getting to it, but we have to follow the breadcrumbs! Leaving out context feels disjointed and incomplete, and interruptions erase our mental whiteboard, forcing us to start over.

This might look like:

- Talking to organize thoughts: "I won't know what I mean until I say it out loud."

- Needing to tell the full story: "If I skip ahead, it won't make sense."

- Getting stuck in details: "I can see the full picture, so I feel like I have to explain all of it."

When you find yourself engaging in verbal processing or narrative thinking:

☑ **Use writing or voice notes** to organize thoughts before a big conversation.

☑ **Lead with the main idea:** "Here's the short version—then I'll explain."

☑ **Let people finish.** If someone processes out loud, interrupting resets their train of thought.

Conversational Timing and Flow

The ADHD brain doesn't always think on command. Sometimes it stalls. Other times it floods your mind with thoughts that weren't even on the radar moments before. One second you're fully engaged in conversation, and the next, a completely unrelated reminder crashes the party—*Don't forget to mail that today.* Just like that, your brain takes a detour.

There are a few reasons why conversational timing gets tricky. First, ADHD brains are sensitive to dopamine. A stimulating conversation can spike dopamine levels, unlocking all kinds of stored thoughts. Second, our brains retrieve by association. A single word can set off a mental domino chain—triggering memories, unrelated ideas, to-do list items, or different topics altogether. It's like your mental inbox flies open and tabs you didn't even know were running pop into view.

These brain-based shifts can throw off your rhythm in a few key ways.

You Interrupt Because You Don't Want to Forget

Your brain works like a dry-erase board—ideas disappear quickly if not written down or spoken out loud. If you don't say it now, it's gone. But holding the thought too tightly can pull you out of the present moment and make it hard to stay engaged with what the other person is saying.

TOOLBOX: Interrupting

- ☑ **Jot down a keyword** on a notepad or in your phone to save the thought.

- ☑ **Mentally tag it** by silently repeating the idea to yourself—but keep listening.

- ☑ **Build in a pause buffer.** Take a breath before jumping in. If you still remember it, it's worth saying.

- ☑ **Name the moment** if you do interrupt: "Sorry, I got excited—go ahead!"

You Lose Track Mid-Conversation

Fast-paced discussions and a lagging mental Wi-Fi signal don't mix. You might still be processing the last sentence while the topic has already changed, or you planned a response while they were talking, only to realize it no longer fits.

TOOLBOX: Losing Track

- ☑ **Mentally summarize** what they just said before responding: "So, you're saying..."

- ☑ **Ask for a quick rewind** with phrases like "That part went over my head—can you repeat it?" or "Let me make sure I got this right..."

- ☑ **Take a processing pause:** "Hang on, I'm catching up," or "Wait—I think I missed something important. Can we go back a second?"

You Go on a Tangent

One idea sparks another and another. Suddenly you're three stories deep and nowhere near the original point. Your ADHD brain loves a good idea trail, but staying on topic can be tough when associations fire faster than filters.

TOOLBOX: Tangents

- ☑ **Circle back gracefully:** "Oops, my brain took a detour. What were we talking about?"

- ☑ **Set a quick anchor** before starting your story: "Here's the short version..." or "Let me back up for context."

Learning to manage the rhythm of conversations isn't about talking less—it's about creating space to stay present and connected while your brilliant brain does its thing. With practice, you'll find a pace that allows your thoughts to land clearly, not just arrive quickly.

Social Recall

ADHD brains don't store social information efficiently. While neurotypical brains tend to categorize names, faces, and interactions like files in a cabinet, ADHD brains process people more like vivid experiences. But once that moment passes, it's like the file gets misplaced—or wiped away like dry-erase marker on a board.

Here are three common ways social recall challenges show up—and how to work with them.

Forgetting Names

While others lock in names, your brain may be focused on someone's energy, clothing, or tone of voice. If the name doesn't register right away, it's often gone.

TOOLBOX: Forgetting Names

- ☑ **Say their name immediately.** When someone introduces themselves, repeat it right away: "Nice to meet you, Sarah! So, Sarah, what do you do?" Repeating it out loud reinforces memory.

- ☑ **Make an association.** Connect their name to a visual or personal detail—"Mark in dark clothes," or "Kelcey from yoga." The stronger the image, the more likely it'll stick.

- ☑ **Keep a people log.** After social events, jot down quick notes: "Met Sam at yoga—two dogs, graphic designer." It's like creating your own external memory bank.

- ☑ **Be honest if you forget.** A simple "I'm great with faces, not so much with names—remind me?" builds connection and models self-compassion.

Forgetting Past Conversations

Your working memory prioritizes what's urgent now, not what happened last week. If you don't anchor the conversation, the memory fades quickly.

TOOLBOX: Forgetting Past Conversations

- ☑ **Anchor details with imagery.** As someone shares something personal, mentally link it to a visual cue: "Joe's kid started soccer" = picture Joe on a field with cleats.

- ☑ **Keep social notes.** After a chat, write down key points: "Alex is moving next month. Stressed about packing." These notes become a cheat sheet you can review before seeing someone again.

☑ **Ask for a recap.** If you're fuzzy on what was said, try: "I remember the topic, but not the details—can you remind me what we said about that?"

Losing Track of Relationships

Without visual reminders, people may slip off your mental map. You may forget to reach out—or accidentally treat a distant acquaintance like a close friend.

TOOLBOX: Losing Track of Relationships

☑ **Set reminders to connect.** Schedule check-ins in your calendar or phone: "Text Dad Sunday," "Check in with Mel after her appointment."

☑ **Categorize people mentally.** When you meet someone, give your brain a folder: "work friend," "coffee shop buddy," "neighbor with the dog." This helps with recall later.

☑ **Use context clues** when you draw a blank. If someone feels familiar but you're unsure, ease into it with:

- "It's so good to see you! Catch me up—what's new?"

- "Remind me, where did we last hang out?"

- "I'm the worst at staying in touch, but I love reconnecting when I do."

Emotional Memory Distortion

Emotional memory distortion is when your brain stores the *feeling* of a conversation, but not the *facts*. Instead of remembering the exact words, you recall the emotional vibe—how something made you feel, not necessarily what was actually said.

This can become a problem when your brain fills in the blanks with its best guess. But those guesses are not always accurate.

If you already feel insecure in social settings, even a neutral moment can spiral into rejection sensitivity (hello, RSD), especially when nothing was actually wrong. You might confidently recall something someone said—except…they didn't. Or you're sure you apologized, but your friend swears you never did.

Our brains are wired to store emotional intensity more than verbal details. You might remember feeling awkward or criticized but not the exact words. You replay a moment over and over, and each time, the details get a little fuzzier. Eventually, your brain fills in what it *thinks* happened—and that's what sticks.

You might also:

- Mix up who said what, or when it happened

- Be convinced a conversation took place that never actually did

- Feel hurt over something that was never meant negatively—but the emotional impression took over

TOOLBOX: Emotional Memory Disortion

- ☑ **Write things down.** If something matters, take notes right after.

- ☑ **Double-check before assuming.** Ask: "Wait, did I actually say that, or just think about saying it?"

- ☑ **Check in with others.** "Hey, I remember feeling weird about that convo, but I can't remember why. Did I miss something?"

- ☑ **Admit when you're unsure.** "I remember feeling like we talked about this, but I might be mixing things up."

If someone corrects your memory, don't get defensive. Just say "Oh, my bad! I must have misremembered." People appreciate that far more than debating it. And it shows that you're self-aware, not careless.

Conclusion

Conversations can be unpredictable, fast-paced, and full of moving parts. Keeping up can feel like navigating a mental obstacle course. Struggling with social working memory doesn't mean you're bad at conversations, it just means your brain processes and organizes information differently.

You don't have to be perfect to connect with others. What matters most is being present, engaged, and giving yourself the grace to navigate interactions in a way that works for *you*.

If you need a second to think, take it.

If you lose your train of thought, circle back.

If you forget something, ask.

If you go on a tangent, own it and redirect.

Most people aren't analyzing your every word—they're too focused on their own experience. So let go of the pressure to get it all right. Conversations aren't about performance; they're about connection.

If you saw yourself in any of the challenges from this chapter, start with just one. Pick a strategy, try it out, and give it space to stick. With time and repetition, small shifts lead to big changes. Before you know it, you'll feel more present, more confident, and more at ease in your conversations.

Chapter 7

Time Management

Some people hang a tennis ball from a string in their garage to avoid driving straight into the wall. For those who struggle with depth perception, that tennis ball is a lifesaver—it keeps them from accidentally parking in their own living room! They can't sense where the car is in relation to the wall, so they rely on that bouncing ball to save the day.

If you struggle with time perception, you need a tennis ball like that, but for your brain. Something to "bop" you on the head just as you're about to lose another forty-five minutes researching whether penguins have knees.

Without good time perception, you might send holiday cards in January, show up for meetings that happened yesterday, or start a college fund the day your kid gets their acceptance letter. Behind, ahead, unprepared—this is life when time feels more like a loose suggestion than a reliable roadmap.

Your brain's internal tennis ball is your *time management executive function*. It helps you be on time, remember important dates, and plan for tomorrow while living in today. And when it comes to your social life, this function helps you follow through on plans, show up when you say you will, and build lasting connections. When it's working, people see you as thoughtful and dependable. When it's not, despite your best intentions, you can come off as scattered, forgetful, or unreliable.

In this chapter, we'll explore two core challenges, *time blindness* and *time nearsightedness*, and four key skills that can help you bring time into focus.

Time Blindness

Time blindness, also known as time agnosia, is the experience of not being able to *feel* time passing. It's not just losing track of a few minutes here or there. It's struggling to estimate how long things take, stick to schedules, or sense where you are in time.

For ADHDers, this is more than a quirky trait. It's a neurological hiccup. You sit down to scroll for what feels like thirty minutes... and suddenly it's been two hours. Or you're stuck in a meeting that feels like it's dragging into next week—but nope, it's only been ten minutes.

Time either flies or crawls, with no reliable rhythm. That's how you end up saying "I'll be back in half an hour!" and walking in the door three hours later. Or feeling frustrated and restless because something that feels endless has barely even started.

So, what's really happening behind the scenes? Why does time feel so slippery, and why does urgency suddenly snap it into focus?

Time and the Nervous System

One of the biggest reasons ADHDers struggle with time is because the ADHD brain doesn't process it logically; it processes it emotionally. Time isn't just about clocks and calendars. It's about chemistry.

Researchers have shown that time distortion in ADHD is tied to dopamine dysregulation (Barkley 1997; Volkow et al. 2009). Dopamine plays a key role in motivation, focus, and time estimation. When it's running low, your sense of time gets foggy.

You might not feel time passing until there's a fire behind you. Then—*boom!*—everything snaps into focus. That's because stress hormones like adrenaline temporarily boost dopamine. Suddenly, you *can* feel time... and the panic too.

This is why many ADHDers live in a loop of delay, panic, and sprint. Urgency works—but only for a while. Running on adrenaline might help you meet the deadline, but it also traps your nervous system in overdrive, leading to burnout.

When your brain is wired for stress, even small tasks can feel overwhelming, or totally invisible until it's nearly too late. And once that pressure hits, hyperfocus isn't far behind.

The good news? You don't have to rely on panic to make time feel real. With the right tools, you can train your brain to notice time *before* it becomes an emergency.

Skills for Sensing Time

Because ADHD brains forget what's out of sight, try hanging a large yearly calendar where you'll see it every day. Mark it with holidays, events, and deadlines. A full-year view helps your brain *feel* where you are in time.

Countdowns can boost urgency. Before my daughter's wedding, "forty-five days" felt way more real than "two months." Same with the holidays—Halloween to Christmas is about fifty-five days, but if your goal is to finish shopping by December first, that's only thirty-one days—or five weekends. Suddenly, it feels a lot closer.

Want to sharpen your time sense? Try the one-minute test: Set a timer, close your eyes, and open them when you think a minute has passed. Then check how close you were. Practicing this can help fine-tune your internal clock.

Skills for Estimating Time

Time estimates often feel like wild guesses, and ADHD guesses tend to miss the mark. You might assume something takes fifteen minutes, only to discover it always takes forty. That gap leads to rushing, unfinished tasks, and a lot of unnecessary stress.

To sharpen your sense of time, try a quick reality check: time your morning routine. Pick one day and track how long each part actually takes—shower, getting dressed, breakfast, packing up. You might think it takes an hour, but it's really an hour and a half. Even timing things once or twice is enough to give your brain a more accurate reference point.

Knowing how long things *really* take helps you plan better, finish what you start, and avoid the last-minute scramble. And that feels good.

Practicing this regularly helps fine-tune your internal clock—especially helpful if your ADHD brain tends to lose track of time. Try it once a week or whenever you want to reconnect with how time *feels*.

Time Nearsightedness

Like nearsighted vision, time nearsightedness means you can focus on what's right in front of you but struggle to see what's further out. Deadlines, plans, and goals in the future might feel vague, distant, or even unreal, until they're suddenly right on top of you.

It's like needing glasses and not realizing it. Everyone else seems to see the future clearly, while you're squinting, trying to make out the shape of things to come. You might feel disorganized, behind, or even ashamed for not being able to plan like others do.

Luckily, there *are* glasses for this. These are skills like reflective foresight and time horizons, which help bring the future into focus. They give your brain the support it needs to connect today's actions with tomorrow's outcomes—so you can plan ahead without the panic.

Reflective Foresight

Reflective foresight means using your past experiences to make smarter plans for the future. Instead of repeating the same "How did this sneak up on me again?" moments, you build in support for future you without the guilt trip.

Here's how to start:

1. **Recall a challenging moment.** Think of a time you felt rushed or unprepared—like doing your taxes at the last minute because you didn't track expenses.

2. **Identify one change goal.** Choose one small improvement for next time, like tracking receipts weekly instead of scrambling in April.

3. **Make it a habit**. Support your goal with a weekly routine. Just ten minutes every Friday can prevent a month of future stress.

4. **Expand to other areas.** Once that habit sticks, apply the same approach to other goals, like setting aside holiday money throughout the year or prepping for birthdays ahead of time.

5. **Look ahead.** Ask yourself regularly, *What would make this easier for future me?* Small changes now can prevent big headaches later.

6. **Notice what worked.** Growth isn't just about fixing mistakes—it's also about building on wins. When something goes smoothly, pause and ask, *What did I do here?* Then do more of that.

Time Horizons

Time horizons help you to anticipate, plan, and prepare for where you're going. Imagine you're a traveler looking out at the horizon. You see landmarks nearby and others farther away, helping you plan your route. In the same way, time horizons let you "map out" your future, helping you decide what steps to take now to reach your long-term goals. Here's how to use a time horizon to plan something like a stress-free dinner party:

1. **Define your destination (the big goal):** You want to host a smooth, enjoyable dinner party. Planning ahead can help avoid last-minute stress.

2. **Set milestones for key tasks:** Break the plan into long-, mid-, and short-term actions:

   • Long-term (a few weeks before): Plan the menu and finalize your guest list.

   • Mid-term (the week before): Shop for ingredients and prep what you can.

- Short-term (the night before): Set the table and finish food prep.

3. **Use reminders and countdowns:** Add key tasks to your calendar and set phone reminders. Numbering the days leading up to the event (e.g., "ten days until dinner party") helps orient you in time and builds a realistic sense of urgency.

4. **Celebrate small wins and adjust as needed:** With each milestone completed, you reduce stress and build momentum. By the time your guests arrive, you'll feel prepared and present—not frazzled.

You can also use this technique when packing for vacations. Instead of a stressful, rushed packing session the night before, start a month in advance. Set out your suitcase and gradually add items, writing down on a notepad the things you need to get as they come to mind. Then, the week of your trip, go through what you've gathered and remove any unnecessary items. This way, you're prepared and can pack without the last-minute rush.

Keeping Relationships in Focus

Like we mentioned in the working memory chapter, even when relationships matter to you, they can slip from your mind once they're not right in front of you. You've probably had moments when you run into someone and suddenly remember, *Oh, I really like them! We should hang out more.* You say, "Let's get together soon!"—but once they're out of sight, the thought disappears again, and nothing happens.

Of course you care about your friends, but time blindness makes it harder to keep relationships in mind. The key is using intentional time management strategies to stay connected.

Turning Intentions into Connection

Keeping relationships strong takes more than good intentions—it takes follow-through. The key is turning fleeting thoughts into planned actions. These small shifts add up to meaningful connection.

☑ **Say it, then schedule it.** When you say, "Let's get together," pull out your phone and book it right then. Add it to your calendar with a reminder so it doesn't slip away.

☑ **Follow up after events.** Jot down names of people you want to reconnect with after a gathering. Then set reminders to reach out. A quick text, email, or call can go a long way.

☑ **Make important dates visible.** Keep birthdays, anniversaries, and life milestones on a calendar you check often. Use reminders or recurring alerts so nothing sneaks past you.

☑ **Plan ahead for special occasions.** Stock up on cards or small gifts in advance. Even having a note ready to send helps you avoid the last-minute scramble and show others they matter.

☑ **Build a relationship rhythm.**

- Set connection goals: Who do you want to stay close to this season?

- Create routines: Weekly texts, monthly coffee dates, seasonal check-ins.

- Use tools: Apps like Marco Polo, Voxer, or scheduled messages can make staying in touch feel easier.

- Review and refresh: Each week, take a minute to look over your list, plan a few meet-ups, and add reminders.

Relationships thrive with intention. A little planning turns "we should hang out" into "I'm so glad we did."

Punctuality and Social Time Awareness

With ADHD, turning good intentions into follow-through is key. Adopting an "early is on time" mindset can make social interactions smoother and less stressful:

☑ **Build in time buffers.** Add a fifteen- to thirty-minute margin before events to account for unexpected delays. For example, if you typically leave at 2:30 p.m. for a 3 p.m. appointment, aim for 2 p.m. instead.

☑ **Use interval alarms.** If you have a habit of getting caught up in tasks before an event, set alarms at intervals (e.g., 7 a.m., 8:45 a.m., and 9 a.m.) to help transition smoothly.

☑ **Avoid last-minute tasks.** Even if you have extra time, resist the urge to squeeze in one more thing. That "quick" task can easily make you late.

Managing Airtime in Conversations

Staying on track in conversations and respecting others' time is key to social time management. Here are some strategies to help:

☑ **Balance the conversation.** If you share about your trip, ask about theirs. A natural back-and-forth keeps both people engaged. Try to speak for two to three minutes before giving the other person space to respond. If needed, glance at a clock or timer to stay on track.

☑ **Check in with your listener.** A simple "Am I making sense?" or "How are we doing on time?" shows you value their engagement and helps keep the conversation balanced.

☑ **Match the flow.** Pay attention to how long others typically talk before switching topics. A five-to-ten-minute window is a good benchmark for casual conversations.

☑ **Use a visual cue.** If you struggle with time blindness, keeping a timer or clock in view can help you stay aware of how long you've been talking.

Practicing these skills helps create smoother, more engaging interactions, making conversations feel more natural and enjoyable for everyone.

Self-Care for Relationship Health

Social connections thrive when they're nurtured, but maintaining relationships shouldn't come at the cost of your well-being. Prioritizing self-care ensures that you can show up for others in a way that feels sustainable, balanced, and fulfilling.

Avoid Overcommitment

Packing your day with back-to-back events might seem productive, but it easily leads to stress and burnout. Leaving gaps between commitments allows time to transition, prepare, and recharge. These "margins" help you enjoy your day rather than just going through the motions.

Avoid Double-Booking

Sometimes FOMO (fear of missing out) gets the best of us, and we double-book because we don't want to miss anything. But juggling multiple plans adds stress and makes it hard to be fully present. You might spend one event distracted by the next, show up late and miss something important, or cancel last minute. This can leave others feeling unimportant. Over time, it chips away at trust and makes people unsure if they can count on you.

It's okay to miss out. When you say no to one thing, you're saying yes to something else. You're choosing better quality time, less stress, and more authentic connection. You're not rejecting others by picking one gathering over another. You're taking care of your relationships by honoring your limits so you can show up, be present, and connect. Try committing to one event at a time. When you do, you send a powerful message: *This moment matters. You matter.* That's what builds lasting, meaningful relationships.

Say No So You Can Say Yes

People with ADHD often want to say yes to everything—especially in the moment, when the excitement is high or someone we care about is asking. But saying yes without checking our bandwidth can lead to last-minute cancellations, resentment, or burnout.

The truth is, saying no is an act of integrity. It keeps you from making promises you can't keep and protects your time, energy, and relationships. A clear "no" is kinder than a "yes" you can't follow through on. Others might not love hearing no, but they'll respect it—especially when it means that your yes really means something.

Try giving yourself a buffer by saying, "Let me check my schedule and get back to you." That pause gives you space to assess your energy and priorities. When you do say yes, it will be from a place of authenticity, not obligation—and that makes all the difference.

Pace Yourself

Pacing social events means balancing your energy. Set a rhythm that alternates between social and personal time, like having one action-filled weekend, then taking the next weekend off for rest and errands. This balance helps you prioritize quality over quantity, keeping you energized and engaged rather than drained.

Next time you're invited somewhere, *pause before answering.* Check your calendar, consider your energy levels, and ask yourself if you really want to go, or if you need to save energy for something else. Saying "Let me check my schedule" gives you space to make a realistic choice.

Avoid Burnout

While social time is important, downtime is essential too. Set specific days for socializing and others for personal activities, hobbies, or rest. This balance helps you stay refreshed, keeps your enthusiasm for social interactions high, and prevents overwhelm.

Conclusion

Just knowing you have time blindness or time nearsightedness is part of the solution. It shifts your mindset from hoping things will fall into place to realizing that "one day" doesn't happen without support. Time blindness and time nearsightedness aren't something you outgrow. Just like being nearsighted or farsighted, you won't wake up with perfect time perception. But just like glasses bring visual clarity, the right tools can bring time into focus.

The key is learning how your brain experiences time—and choosing strategies that work with it. Internal time awareness is often unreliable, but external tools like calendars, alarms, and reminders help bridge the gap. Instead of relying on memory to follow up or meet deadlines, use structure to help keep what matters in view.

Expecting yourself to always be on time isn't realistic. Life isn't that predictable, and neither are we. Give yourself grace when things don't go as planned. Time may never feel natural, but with the right support, you can move through it intentionally, showing up when it counts, creating space for what matters, and building a life that aligns with your values. Because in the end, your worth isn't measured by a clock, but by the heart you bring to each moment.

Chapter 8

Strategic Communication

You're upset and need to talk to your partner. You start venting every thought, every feeling, every detail. After a long, winding rant, they look at you and ask, "So...what's your point? What do you want?" And honestly? You're not even sure anymore.

Welcome to ADHD-style communication, where you have a lot to say, but your actual message is buried somewhere under a landslide of emotions, tangents, and half-formed thoughts. Strategic communication is about digging that message out. In this chapter, we'll explore how to organize your thoughts, figure out what really matters, and express yourself in a way that actually lands.

By the end, you'll have tools to turn mental clutter into clear, intentional conversations, especially in your relationships.

Communication Challenges

ADHD adds unique hurdles that can make even simple conversations feel like an uphill climb. Racing thoughts and mid-sentence derailments can make conversations feel scattered or incomplete. Here are some common ways ADHD can make communication more difficult:

- Thoughts move faster than words, making it hard to stay on track

- Tangents and distractions pull the conversation in different directions

- Forgetting your point mid-sentence leaves conversations feeling incomplete

- Impulsivity leads to speaking before organizing thoughts

Priorities vs. Demands

Before you can express what you need, you have to know what matters most. That's harder than it sounds, especially in relationships, where your priorities often bump up against someone else's expectations.

This tug-of-war between what you want and what others need from you is one of the biggest sources of conflict in relationships. Navigating it well means being able to clarify your own priorities and flexibly negotiate when demands compete.

Let's define a few key terms:

- *Priorities* are what *you* care about—the tasks, goals, or responsibilities that matter to you.

- *Demands* are what others ask of you—their priorities, their needs, their requests for your time and energy.

Most people find this balance tricky, but for adults with ADHD, it's even harder. Executive functioning challenges can make it difficult to assess what truly needs attention, sort through mental clutter, and clearly express what you need.

So how do you identify what actually matters to you, especially when it's buried under stress or frustration?

What Protests Say

Let's start with a story.

Joel had been looking forward to working on a personal project. Then his wife, Christine, got a last-minute invite to a networking event and asked if he could watch the kids. He shifted his plans, thinking he'd make up for it the next day—but the next day brought another request. This pattern continued until Joel snapped, accusing her of being selfish. But beneath the protest was a simple need: "I want time for my priorities too."

When we're frustrated, we often lead with complaints instead of clarity. The message gets lost in the emotion. Instead of saying what we need, we say what's wrong.

The trick? Listen for the *need* behind the protest. Here are a few examples:

- Protest: "You never listen to me."

- Request: "I want to feel heard and understood."

- Protest: "You never make time for me."

- Request: "I want to feel connected. I need a night with just us."

When you catch yourself venting, pause and ask:

- *What is this frustration really telling me I need?*

- *If this problem magically disappeared, what would be different?*

- *What would "better" look like?*

This shift moves you from reactivity to clarity—an essential step toward healthy communication.

Wants vs. Shoulds

Once you've named a few priorities, it helps to break them down into two categories:

- *Wants* are things you *choose* because they bring joy, purpose, or fulfillment.

- *Shoulds* are things you *feel obligated* to do—responsibilities, deadlines, or expectations.

When your life leans too far into wants, the practical stuff piles up. But when it tilts too far toward shoulds, you risk burnout, resentment, or feeling like you're just checking boxes without meaning.

These next two tools help you zoom out, sift through noise, and make decisions based on what really matters—to *you*.

The 5-5-5 Rule

This quick tool helps you assess urgency and impact. When you're torn on a task, ask yourself:

Will this matter in five minutes?

If the answer is probably not, it's likely a small stressor.

Will this matter in five days?

If yes, maybe it's worth considering.

Will this matter in five years?

If yes, it's a true priority. Pay attention.

This rule gives perspective, so you're not making big decisions based on momentary stress.

Value Compass

This strategy helps cut through distractions and emotional impulses by aligning decisions with your core values rather than short-term pressures. When torn between tasks or requests, ask:

- *Does this align with my long-term goals?*

- *Am I saying yes out of obligation or because this genuinely matters to me?*

This approach keeps priorities rooted in personal meaning and prevents you from just reacting to external demands.

Riley's Story

Riley's story below shows how these two tools might be applied.

Riley has been feeling overwhelmed. Their boss asked them to take on an extra project at work, their best friend wants them to help plan a last-minute birthday party, and they've been meaning to start a workout routine.

They feel pulled in too many directions: They want to be a good employee and friend. Those are priorities for them. Self-care is also a priority, and they want to be in better health. They want to avoid disappointing anyone, so they think they should say yes to everything.

Step 1: Riley applies the 5-5-5 rule and asks themself:

- Will this matter in 5 minutes?
  - *If they say yes, they'll feel immediate relief from avoiding guilt.*
  - *But they know that feeling won't last.*

- Will this matter in 5 days?
  - *The work project will still be there and could lead to added stress if they take it on without bandwidth.*
  - *Their friend's party will be over, and while it's important to celebrate, will their presence or absence make or break their friendship?*
  - *Skipping workouts will add up, making it harder to start a new habit.*

- Will this matter in 5 years?

    - *If they take on too much, they might burn out or feel resentful.*

    - *Strengthening relationships matters in the long term but helping plan one party might not be the deciding factor.*

    - *Their health and well-being matter most over time, meaning their workout routine shouldn't always be the first thing they sacrifice.*

Looking at the big picture, Riley realized that they don't have to say yes to everything just because it feels urgent in the moment. Their desire to be a good employee and friend is still important, even if they occasionally need to say no.

Step 2: To double-check their process, Riley reflects on their core values: *balance, well-being, and meaningful relationships.* They ask themself, *What priorities align with my long-term goals?*

- *Taking care of their health is part of their long-term well-being, so prioritizing their workout is a commitment to themselves.*

- *Doing quality work at their job is important, but only when it does not come at the expense of their mental health.*

- *Supporting their friend is valuable, but that does not mean they have to take on all the planning.*

With their priorities in order, Riley decides:

- *They will not take on the extra work project and will explain to their boss that they do not have the bandwidth right now.*

- *They will help with one small part of the party but will set a boundary about how much they can contribute.*

- *They will prioritize their workout because long-term health matters more than short-term guilt.*

*By making conscious decisions instead of reacting to pressure,
Riley protects their well-being while still supporting others. The
5-5-5 rule helps Riley sort urgency from true importance. Using
their values as a guide allows them to set boundaries without guilt.*

Inflexibility

While some people struggle with saying no, the opposite problem—
being too rigid in priorities—can also happen. If you find yourself feeling
frustrated when things don't go as planned or are struggling to shift gears
when unexpected demands arise, the issue may be difficulties with adaptability and flexibility.

Impairments in cognitive adaptability can make it difficult to:

- Adjust plans when new information or changes arise

- Handle interruptions without feeling thrown off course

- Shift between tasks or priorities without frustration

- Compromise in relationships without feeling like you're
  "losing"

If this sounds familiar, you might notice that you hold tightly to your
own priorities, sometimes to the point of resisting negotiation or compromise. While protecting your own needs is important, rigidly sticking to
plans without considering external factors can create conflict, frustration, and resentment in relationships.

Organizing Thoughts

When organizing thoughts is difficult, conversations can feel scattered or
overwhelming. Using structured techniques can improve clarity and
flow. Before you start a conversation, try using a few of the following
tools to focus your message.

THINK

Before speaking, it helps to slow down and organize your thoughts. The THINK method provides a quick, structured way to clarify what you want to say before you say it:

Topic—What's the main idea I need to focus on?

Heart—What's the core message I want to communicate?

Important details—What supporting points are necessary?

Not necessary—What details can I leave out to avoid confusion?

Key takeaway—What do I want the other person to remember?

This framework helps filter out unnecessary information, keeping the conversation focused.

The One-Sentence Rule

Before speaking, try summarizing your main point in one clear sentence. If you can't, take a moment to organize your thoughts. Be specific and leave out filler words and add-ons. Instead of saying,

"I was thinking maybe we should figure out the thing we were supposed to do because I know it's due soon, but I also have another idea I wanted to bring up."
Try,

"We need to finalize the project plan today so we stay on track."
Leading with clarity helps the listener stay engaged and understand your message faster.

Mind Mapping

This visual tool helps structure thoughts before speaking:

1. Write the main topic in the center of a page.

2. Branch out into key points related to the topic.

3. Add supporting details under each point.

Mind mapping is useful for planning discussions, structuring arguments, and reducing mental clutter.

Communicating Clearly

Effective communication starts with organizing your thoughts (using some of the strategies you just read about). The next step is expressing them in a way that others can easily understand. By using simple strategies, you can stay focused, reduce misunderstandings, and feel more confident in conversations.

Clarifying the Purpose

Many people talk for different reasons: sometimes to vent and feel heard, sometimes to sort out their thoughts, and sometimes to find a solution. But if the listener doesn't know what you need, they might respond in a way that frustrates you instead of helping. A simple way to avoid this is by clarifying the purpose of the conversation upfront.

If you're the listener, you can ask:

"Do you want me to just listen, help you organize your thoughts, or help you find a solution?"

If you're the one talking, try saying:

"Hey, I need to talk about something. Right now, I just need to vent—can you just listen and tell me what you hear?"

or

"I'm trying to figure something out, and I could use your help finding a solution."

This small change prevents miscommunication, frustration, and mismatched expectations, making conversations more productive and supportive.

Beginning, Middle, and End

Do you ever start talking and realize mid-sentence you don't know where you're going? Or maybe you jump from topic to topic, leaving your listener confused? Structuring what you say with a clear beginning, middle, and end helps keep conversations focused and engaging.

The Beginning: Set It Up

Start with a quick introduction so the listener knows where you're going:

- "I had a situation at work today that reminded me of what we talked about last week."

- "There's something on my mind, and I'd love your thoughts."

This grabs attention and keeps the listener engaged.

The Middle: Give Key Details

Stick to relevant details and avoid unnecessary tangents. Instead of,

"So my boss gave me two projects, and I was already behind because of that meeting yesterday, and anyway, I was thinking about what we said last week..."
try,

"My boss gave me two big assignments at once, and I felt completely overwhelmed."

The End: Wrap It Up

Summarize, ask a question, or make a request:

- "That's why I wanted to ask—how do you handle situations like that?"

- "Anyway, it made me realize I need to set better boundaries at work."

If you need to be very concise, you can shorten this method into three short sentences:

1. Intro (What's the point?): "I had a stressful situation at work today."

2. Middle (Why does it matter?): "My boss gave me two major assignments at once, and I felt overwhelmed."

3. End (What's the takeaway?): "How would you handle that?"

Using a beginning, middle, and end keeps conversations clear, concise, and easy to follow. Instead of losing your point, you'll express yourself in a way that's structured, intentional, and engaging.

Conclusion

Strategic communication is about intention, organizing your thoughts, clarifying your needs, and expressing yourself in ways others can understand. It's about knowing what matters to you, understanding what matters to others, and navigating that space with clarity, adaptability, flexibility, and self-respect.

But strategy doesn't mean rigidity. Life is messy, and conversations don't always follow a script. That's where flexibility comes in—being able to adjust without losing yourself.

Start small. Choose one strategy from this chapter and try it in a low-pressure moment. With practice, it won't just feel easier, it'll start to flow like a pro.

Chapter 9

Perspective-Taking and Attunement

Let's say you're hanging out with friends, and someone tells a story about getting stuck in an elevator for two hours. You jump in with, "That reminds me of the time I had to pee in a bottle on a road trip!"

Your friend looks at you, horrified. You notice the awkward silence three beats too late. Then, about seven hours later, it hits you: *Ohhh. They weren't looking for a bathroom disaster story. They were talking about feeling claustrophobic and scared. I missed that completely! No wonder they looked at me like that!*

If you've ever been labeled as insensitive or oblivious, take a breath. It may not be that you don't care—it may just be that your nervous system doesn't serve up social insights as fast as everyone else's. Your brain takes the scenic route to figuring it out.

That's where *perspective-taking* and *attunement* come in. Perspective-taking is an executive function skill that helps you understand what someone else might be thinking or feeling. Attunement is your ability to notice and respond to what's happening in the moment, like reading a room or recognizing when someone's getting upset.

In this chapter, we'll explore both. By the end, you'll have practical tools to:

- Spot perspective-taking blind spots in real time (not hours later)

- Adjust your energy without masking who you are

- Turn social cringes into connection wins

So, buckle up—because understanding how others think (and how you come across) doesn't have to be a mystery. This chapter will give you the tools to navigate social moments with more insight, ease, and connection.

What Is Perspective-Taking?

Perspective-taking is the ability to step outside your own viewpoint and consider someone else's experience. even if it's totally different from yours. It's what helps us understand where someone is coming from, avoid misunderstandings, and foster empathy (even if we don't agree).

At its core, perspective-taking is about seeing the big picture and understanding that the same situation can be experienced completely differently by others. Imagine two people on a roller coaster. One is laughing; the other is passed out. Without perspective-taking, the excited friend assumes the other loved it too—then argues when they say, "That was awful!"

For ADHDers, this skill can be especially tricky. Emotional intensity, black-and-white thinking, or taking things personally can cloud our ability to see the bigger picture. But with practice, we can learn to pause and ask: *What else might be going on here?*

Perspective-taking helps you:

- Recognize others' emotional states

- Adjust your communication to meet people where they are

- Consider other explanations before jumping to conclusions

We all interpret the world through our own lens, and that self-bias can make it harder to recognize that someone else might see the same situation very differently, especially when emotions are running high.

For those of us with ADHD, that lens can be even more skewed. Intense emotions, rejection sensitivity, and fast-moving thoughts can make it easy to take things personally or miss the bigger picture.

Try asking: *What might I not be seeing about their experience?*

- When someone doesn't text back: Instead of assuming they're ignoring you, perspective-taking helps you brainstorm other possibilities—maybe their phone died, they're overwhelmed, or they simply need time to respond.

- When someone snaps at you: Perhaps they're tired, or stressed and it wasn't about you.

Reactions are complex and shaped by emotional state, past experiences, and individual processing styles. Even when someone's response feels directed at you, it's often more about what's happening inside them.

Mind-Reading vs. Perspective-Taking

Social interactions can sometimes feel like trying to solve a mystery with half the clues missing. You catch a weird look, an awkward silence drags on, or someone says "I'm fine" when their tone says otherwise. If you have ADHD, you might struggle with knowing what to do in these moments. As we've discussed earlier, the ADHD brain doesn't like missing pieces—it's wired to fill in the blanks. But when you don't have enough context, those mental "guesses" can backfire.

That's where mind-reading sneaks in—a common thinking error where you assume you already know what someone else is thinking or feeling, when you probably don't.

We often hear the phrase "Put yourself in someone else's shoes," but there's a big difference between imagining what someone *might* be experiencing and assuming you know for sure. The first is perspective-taking, a skill you can strengthen. The second is mind-reading, and that one tends to stir up misunderstanding and unnecessary drama.

Mind-Reading (Guessing, Reacting)	Perspective-Taking (Checking)
Assumes thoughts without evidence	Considers multiple possibilities
They must be mad at me.	*Maybe they're distracted or busy.*
Reacts emotionally to assumptions	Checks for context before responding
Often leads to anxiety and miscommunication	Improves relationships and reduces conflict

For ADHD brains, fast thinking can be a double-edged sword. That instinct to fill in gaps quickly can lead to assumptions that *feel* true but aren't. Mind-reading happens when you believe that your thoughts are truths and feelings are facts. Instead, perspective-taking invites you to pause and wonder: *What are the facts or am I filling in the blanks?* If you're unsure, check in gently: "Hey, you seemed quiet earlier—everything okay?"

Building Perspective-Taking Skills

Understanding someone else's point of view doesn't always come naturally, especially when your brain is wired to react quickly or fill in the blanks. These next tools will help you to strengthen your ability to see beyond your own experience.

We first introduced the idea of personal culture in chapter 1 to help reduce judgment. Now, we'll build on that concept as a tool for improving perspective-taking.

Recognize Different Personal Cultures

Perspective-taking becomes easier when you remember that everyone operates from their own personal culture—a unique set of social norms, habits, and expectations shaped by their upbringing, environment, neurotype, and values.

I learned this firsthand with a childhood friend. In my family, important guests were welcomed at home and shared meals with us. That was our personal culture—hosting meant closeness. So, whenever I returned to my hometown, I expected her to invite me over to her house. But she always suggested meeting somewhere else. I started to wonder if she really wanted to see me or if she was just being polite.

Eventually, I checked in. It turned out that in her personal culture, special guests were taken *out* somewhere special, while home was reserved for family. Her invitations weren't intended to distance me; she was trying to honor me. Without that conversation, a misread cultural norm might've ended our friendship.

So next time something feels off, ask yourself:

- *What if this is a personal cultural difference?*

- *What would happen if I asked instead of assumed?*

When you approach differences with curiosity instead of judgment, you create space for understanding. It's not about excusing problematic or harmful behavior—it's about pausing long enough to consider that someone else's "normal" might just be different from yours. And in that pause, connection becomes possible.

Pause Before Reacting

When someone's behavior confuses or upsets you, press pause before jumping to conclusions. Ask yourself:

- *What might they be feeling right now?*

- *Could they be going through something hard?*

- *Is there another possible explanation for their behavior?*

Taking this moment to reflect doesn't mean excusing poor behavior —it just helps you respond from curiosity instead of reactivity.

Checking In vs. Assuming

Imagine you reluctantly agree to attend an event at a friend's request. When you arrive, you spot her across the room and wave—but she gives you a blank look and quickly turns away. You think, *Is she ignoring me? Did I do something wrong?*

Before slipping out, you decide to check in. As you approach, she lights up. You say, "Hey! I waved earlier but couldn't tell if you saw me, so I came to say hi." She laughs and says, "Oh my gosh, I'm so glad you're here! My contact popped out and I can't see a thing. I'll need you to be my eyes!"

Moments like this remind us: *checking in* beats jumping to conclusions.

Try questions like these to check in:

- "You seemed a little off earlier—everything okay?"

- "I want to make sure I understood—did you mean...?"

One simple question can replace hours of overthinking.

Practice Empathy

Empathy brings perspective-taking to life. It helps you connect with someone else's emotional experience by showing that you're present, listening, and that their feelings make sense. This builds trust, deepens connection, and makes conversations feel safe and supportive.

One simple way to practice empathy is through reflective statements. These mirror what the other person is expressing without judgment or advice. You don't have to solve their problem—just show them that you get it.

Try saying:

- "That sounds really frustrating."

- "I can see how that would be overwhelming."

- "It makes sense you'd feel that way."

Reflective statements help others feel seen and heard—but empathy doesn't stop there. Communication also means *tuning in* to emotional cues and adjusting your energy or approach in the moment. That's where *attunement* comes in.

Attunement

One day, I was in session with a client who told a hilarious story, and we were doubled over in laughter. When the session ended, I was still smiling as I greeted my next client.

But the moment the door opened, everything shifted. She walked in hunched over, tears streaming down her face. Her pain filled the room.

I knew I needed to meet her there. I took a deep breath, softened my expression, quieted my voice, and let my posture relax. I genuinely cared and I wanted my face, voice, and body to reflect that. My energy adjusted naturally as I focused fully on her pain and what she needed at that moment.

Attunement is the ability to be emotionally present and adjust your energy to meet someone where they are. It's how we say "I see you, and I'm with you"—without words. If someone is sad, attunement means slowing down, softening your tone, and sitting with them in that moment, rather than trying to cheer them up or fix it.

Without attunement, people often feel unseen or dismissed. Imagine:

- A friend shares that they lost their dream job, and someone responds by talking about their promotion

- Someone is grieving, and another person announces their pregnancy

- A coworker is overwhelmed, and someone asks them to take on more

Missing these emotional cues can create distance, even when it's unintentional.

Attunement is about noticing subtle signals, adjusting your presence, and responding in ways that build trust and connection. In the next section, we'll look at five ways to strengthen attunement so you can show up with intention, read emotional cues more accurately, and respond in ways that help others feel safe, seen, and supported.

Bids for Connection

Psychologists John and Julie Gottman (2018) describe *bids for connection* as attempts to engage emotionally, physically, or socially. Bids can be direct, like sharing a story, or subtle, like making eye contact. They are ways of saying "I want to connect with you."

Common bids for connection include:

- Talking, texting, calling, or sending a meme

- Sharing a story or photo and hoping for a response

- Inviting someone to do something together

- Expressing an emotion: "I'm so frustrated" or "Today was great!"

- Using touch: a hug, a tap on the shoulder

- Standing nearby or laughing at a joke

People typically respond in one of three ways: turning toward, turning away, or turning against. Take the bid "Want to grab lunch this weekend?"

- *Turning toward:* "I'd love to! Let's plan something."

- *Turning away:* No response, or distracted silence.

- *Turning against:* "Why would I want to do that? I'm busy."

Turning toward means acknowledging the bid with eye contact, a nod, a touch, or a genuine reply. It strengthens connection and deepens trust. Turning away happens when bids are ignored or dismissed, often unintentionally, due to distraction or preoccupation. Over time, this can create emotional distance. Turning against actively rejects the bid, often with criticism or defensiveness, which damages trust.

Bids aren't always direct or obvious and can be easy to miss, especially when your attention is pulled elsewhere. One day, my son walked up to me while I was working at the dining room table. "Hey Mom, today..." As I looked at him, I got distracted by his teeth and quickly responded, "Did you brush your teeth?" He let out a frustrated sigh and said, "Never mind," then walked away feeling dismissed. Instead of turning toward his bid, I had a turning away response. These reactions are usually unintentional and happen when someone is distracted or preoccupied. I wasn't rejecting or dismissing him on purpose—I was simply focused elsewhere (hello, ADHD), and I missed the emotional cue.

Thankfully, I caught myself and apologized: "I'm sorry. I really do want to hear about your day. What were you saying?"

We all miss bids sometimes. That's okay. Our goal is awareness and the ability to attend to our relationships. When you notice a missed bid, you can turn back toward connection and repair.

Reading the Room

Reading the room means tuning in to the emotional atmosphere and adjusting your energy, tone, and presence to match. It helps you sync with what others are feeling, whether it's a celebration, a tough moment, or something in between, by regulating your energy so that you don't come in too hot or too flat but instead match the mood of the moment.

A key way you can attune to others is through mirroring—the unconscious or intentional matching of someone's facial expressions, tone, and body language. Mirroring helps people feel seen and understood, and it strengthens emotional connection. For example, when someone is visibly upset, speaking in a soft voice and relaxing your posture can help them feel safe and supported. If they're excited, you might lean in, smile, or match their enthusiasm with your own energy. When a friend shares good news and you light up with them, that's mirroring. When a loved one is grieving and you simply sit quietly beside them, offering your presence without pressure, that's mirroring too. These small, subtle shifts signal "I'm here with you." Because attunement is about reading and responding to social cues in real time, mirroring naturally emerges as part of this process.

Body Language

Body language gives subtle clues about how someone is feeling, even when they're not saying anything directly. If someone shifts from looking engaged to seeming checked out or tense, it might be a sign to pause, shift gears, or check in. While body language isn't an exact science, paying attention to it can help you stay better attuned in conversations.

Some common cues include:

- Engagement—eye contact, leaning in, nodding, smiling

- Disengagement—looking away, fidgeting, crossing arms, turning slightly

- Eager to speak—leaning forward, raising a hand or finger, parting their lips as if about to jump in

If you're not sure what someone's body language means, don't panic or assume the worst. Try a quick reality check like:

- "Would you like me to keep going?"

- "You okay? Want me to pause?"

- "I can't tell if I'm rambling—are we good?"

These small moments of curiosity help create attuned two-way dialogue that honors the other person's emotional state and shows you care about their experience, not just your own words.

Voice and Facial Expression

Facial expressions and tone of voice reveal emotions that words don't always capture. When you tune in to these cues, you can better understand how someone's feelings and respond in ways that feel supportive instead of overwhelming. This chart offers common cues and examples of how to adjust your presence in a way that builds connection:

State	Cues to Look For	How to Adjust
Open, Social, or Engaged	Relaxed posture, eye contact, natural smiles, conversational flow	Stay open, engage naturally, match their energy
Overwhelmed, Alert, or On Edge	Fidgeting, fast speech, interrupting, tense expression	Slow down, soften tone, give space to talk
Shut Down or Agitated	Avoiding eye contact, flat or tense face, withdrawn body language	Lower intensity, offer warmth, don't push conversation

Attunement means listening with your eyes and ears, not just your brain, and making small adjustments to meet others where they are.

Timing

Timing shapes how conversations flow. Being attuned to timing means engaging in ways that feel natural rather than rushed, delayed, or disruptive. Here are a few things to watch for:

- ☑ **When to speak or pause:** Notice the flow of conversation. Give space after someone finishes a thought instead of jumping in too quickly.

- ☑ **Choosing the right moment:** Match the mood. A vent session might not be the best time to share exciting news, and a light conversation may not be ready for something heavy.

☑ **Letting the conversation breathe:** If emotions run high or a topic feels exhausted, it may be time to pause or gently change direction instead of pushing through.

☑ **Respecting processing time:** Some people need a few extra seconds to respond. Silence isn't awkward—it's part of thoughtful communication.

Well-timed responses help conversations feel smoother, more respectful, and more connected.

Validation

Validation helps people feel seen, heard, and understood without requiring agreement. It bridges the gap between understanding someone's perspective and connecting with them emotionally. Without validation, conversations can feel dismissive or turn into debates. With it, we build trust, reduce defensiveness, and prevent those "you just don't get it" moments. Effective validation involves the following three steps:

Step 1: I see you. Match their emotional state with your facial expression and tone.

Validation starts before you even speak. It begins with your presence, your face, your voice, your body language. If they're sharing something painful, let your face show concern. If they're joyful, reflect that joy. It's about attuning to their emotional energy and mirroring it with care.

Do: Mirror their emotion. If they are sad, look concerned. If they smile, smile back.

Don't: Mismatch emotions—like smiling when someone is crying. People often do this with good intentions, thinking it will help the other person feel better. But trying to shift someone's mood usually doesn't work. In fact, it can make them feel more upset because it signals you don't understand or aren't truly with them in their emotion.

Step 2: I hear you. Rephrase what you heard to show you're listening and to check for accuracy.

> *Do:* Summarize their words in your own language, then ask, "Did I get that right?" Keep your tone warm and curious.

> *Don't:* Skip the understanding step. Many people respond too quickly—by defending themselves, offering advice, correcting details, or sharing their own experience. But when you do that before showing you truly understand, the other person may feel dismissed or unseen. Validation comes first, then you can offer your response.

> For example:

> *Them:*   You always cut me off when I talk.

> *You:*   Yeah… I do that sometimes. It must feel like I'm not really giving you space to speak. Is that what you mean?

Step 3: I get it. Show empathic understanding.

Validation isn't about agreeing. It's about getting where they're coming from by putting yourself in their shoes. This step focuses on the *feeling* behind the words, not whether their perception is *right* or *wrong*.

> *Do:* Pause and ask yourself, *If that happened to me, how would I feel?* Physically show you are reflecting—like The Thinker statue: hand on chin, looking up, pausing to process. Then reflect that emotion back.

> *Don't:* Argue the facts, jump in with your side of the story, or communicate judgment—like saying "That's ridiculous!"

> For example:

> *Them:*   You never listen to me in meetings.

> *You:*   (*Pause, reflect, then respond with empathy.*) Dang, that would really bug me too. I'd feel like, "Why

even bother talking if no one's hearing me?" Is that kind of how it's been feeling for you?

Sometimes, you might struggle to understand why someone feels the way they do, especially if you'd react differently in their shoes. That's okay. Empathy doesn't always mean *feeling the same*, but it does mean *being willing to try.*

If you genuinely can't connect to the emotion, try this instead:

- ☑ **Be curious and open:** "I want to understand—can you tell me more about what that felt like for you?"

- ☑ **Acknowledge their experience:** "I can see this is really affecting you."

- ☑ **Validate the emotion, even if you don't relate to the situation:** "I don't fully get it, but I can tell it's really upsetting—and that matters to me."

The goal is to create a safe space where the other person feels heard, even if you have different perspectives and experiences.

Now let's take attunement one step further: supporting someone else's regulation through your own. That's the heart of coregulation.

Coregulation

Ever walked into a room and instantly felt calmer or more tense, even if no one said anything? That's emotional contagion. Our nervous systems pick up on each other's cues like tuning forks. It's subtle, automatic, and surprisingly powerful. We sync up without even trying.

That's what coregulation is. It's how nervous systems communicate with each other beneath the surface. According to polyvagal theory, we don't regulate alone—we regulate in connection with others. When someone offers calm, grounded energy, it sends a signal of safety that helps the other person shift out of fight, flight, or freeze. And when you're the calm one in the room, you become the anchor. The steady presence their nervous system can settle into.

Why it matters:

- It reduces tension and creates emotional safety

- It builds trust without needing to fix anything

- It helps communication flow better

- It keeps you steady while supporting someone else

- It helps rewire what connection feels like, especially for people with ADHD or trauma

Coregulation works both ways. If someone is anxious or spiraling, your nervous system might start to pick up on that and go along for the ride. But when you notice it, you have a choice. You can meet them where they are, or you can offer a calmer energy for them to tune in to.

How to Coregulate

If someone near you is anxious, overwhelmed, or upset, your job isn't to fix it. Your job is to regulate yourself first.

☑ **Take a slow breath.**

☑ **Soften your face.**

☑ **Relax your shoulders.**

☑ **Let your body speak safety.**

Your calm presence sends a message without needing words: "I'm with you. You're safe."

Resist the urge to jump in with quick reassurances like "Don't be upset" or "You're fine." They may sound comforting, but to the nervous system they're just noise. The modern brain might understand the words, but the body doesn't buy it. Your nervous system speaks a different language. It responds to what you embody, not what you say. *Tone. Eye contact. Breath. Stillness.*

That's the real power of coregulation. It's not about making someone feel better. It's about showing them they're not alone. It says, "I can stay with you in this moment" and "You're not bad for feeling this way. You're still okay with me." And that's what helps quiet shame.

Coregulation is a quiet kind of magic. As you learned in chapters 2 and 3, neuroception is always scanning for cues of safety. When the nervous system finds those cues, it often shifts out of distress very quickly, like turning on a light in a dark room. The light doesn't fight the darkness, it just illuminates the space.

If you want to help someone regulate, start by being the calm they can lean on. Let your nervous system go first.

Conclusion

Perspective-taking helps you zoom out, attunement helps you zoom in, and the regulation skills you've learned in previous chapters help you stay steady while doing both. Together, they create a kind of social fluency— a flexible, grounded way of connecting with others—even when the moment is emotionally charged or unclear.

When you can see others clearly, meet them where they are, and stay anchored in your own nervous system, you open the door to genuine connection. These skills don't require perfection. They just ask for presence, curiosity, and willingness.

Instead of spiraling about what someone meant, you check in.

Instead of shrinking after a misstep, you repair.

Instead of masking or overthinking, you adjust with authenticity.

So when things feel messy, uncertain, or awkward:

Ask instead of assume.

Breathe instead of brace.

And keep showing up—open, present, and connected.

Chapter 10

Who Told You That?

Maybe no one ever said it outright. Maybe it was the eye rolls, the sighs, or the way people pulled away when you got excited. A teacher who sighed when you raised your hand. A parent who scolded you for talking too fast or moving too slow. A boss, partner, or friend who made you feel like being yourself was a problem. Somewhere along the way, you got the message: You're too much.

With ADHD, you've likely internalized negative feedback over time, carrying its weight long into adulthood. But what if that feedback was wrong? Who made them the authority on what's "too much"? People have different preferences, tolerances, and capacities. What overwhelms one person might energize another.

You can't control people's opinions, but you can control how much space they take up in your mind.

In this chapter, you'll learn how to:

- Distinguish helpful feedback from harmful feedback so you stop owning things that aren't yours

- Recognize safe vs. unsafe people

- Spot manipulation tactics that can leave you second-guessing yourself

- Recognize healthy and unhealthy boundaries

Learning to trust yourself, navigate relationships with clarity, and set firm boundaries takes practice. But once you stop handing your power over to others, you reclaim it for yourself and step into self-leadership.

Let's dive in.

Self-Blame

Self-blame is one of the sneakiest survival strategies we develop as kids. It doesn't always make sense to blame ourselves for things that weren't our fault. But in chaotic environments, self-blame creates an illusion of control:

- *If the problem is me, maybe I can fix it.*

- *If I just behave better, maybe they won't get angry.*

- *If I can anticipate their needs perfectly, maybe I won't be abandoned.*

Letting go of control is a whole other book. For now, we can acknowledge that while there's a lot we can't control, we *can* take action to prevent self-blame.

Discernment

As a kid, you probably didn't think much about the feedback you received. Without the tools to question whether it was fair or healthy, you likely took it to heart if adults told you something was wrong with you.

When those messages kept coming, you started to form an idea of who you are, measuring your worth by how well you met others' expectations. Over time, your sense of self wasn't just based on who you are—it was shaped by how others saw you.

That's why, as an adult, every critique might still feel like a gut punch. Every opinion may seem like the truth, and trusting your own judgment might feel foreign because no one ever gave you permission to trust yourself.

The good news? You can learn to separate feedback that helps you grow from the stuff that just weighs you down. Not all feedback is created equal. Some is constructive and helps you grow, while some is misguided or biased, making you second-guess yourself when you don't need to.

Filtering feedback is a skill, and like any skill, it takes practice. Ask yourself:

- *Is it valid or based on assumptions?*

- *Is it specific and constructive, or vague and judgmental?*

- *Does it align with what I know to be true about myself?*

- *Does this person have expertise in this area? Are they familiar with ADHD or are they seeing it through a neurotypical lens?*

- *Do I trust and respect their opinion?*

Just because someone influenced you in the past doesn't mean they should still define how you see yourself today. If you wouldn't let them make decisions for you now, why let their words hold power over you?

Sometimes, writing feedback down and reading it as if it were about someone else can provide clarity. Ask yourself: *Does this feedback help me grow?*

- Constructive feedback offers actionable solutions, like "You might try organizing your tasks differently."

- Harmful feedback is vague, judgmental, and shaming, like "You're lazy and irresponsible."

Not every opinion deserves your energy. The next time someone gives you unsolicited feedback, remember, you get to decide whether to accept it or leave it unread and unbothered.

And when harmful feedback keeps coming from the same people? It's time to ask: Is this person safe, or should they be reconsidered in your life?

Safe vs. Unsafe People

Healthy relationships are built on mutual respect, trust, and emotional safety. In these kinds of connections, you don't have to prove your worth, earn kindness, or constantly adjust just to keep the peace.

But it can be tricky to tell the difference between safe and unsafe people. ADHDers, especially, tend to connect quickly. We're often drawn to the excitement or intensity of shared emotional experiences, rather than long-term trustworthiness. Plus, fear of rejection might make us more willing to tolerate unsafe behaviors just to avoid conflict.

On top of that, ADHD can mess with our ability to track long-term patterns in relationships. It can be harder to notice subtle shifts in respect, responsibility, or reciprocity, especially when our working memory is in overdrive trying to juggle everything.

If you've found yourself stuck in toxic relationships, it's important to remember: it's not your fault. But you do have the power to change it. Learning to trust your gut, set boundaries without guilt, and recognize unhealthy patterns are the first steps in building healthier, more fulfilling connections.

Understanding what to look for can help you decide which relationships to nurture, and which ones may need distance. (You can find a table of characteristics of safe vs. unsafe people in the online materials at http://www.newharbinger.com/56166.)

Action over Words

Be cautious of people who *tell you* who they are instead of showing you. Someone who constantly declares "I'm a loyal friend" or "You can trust me" but acts in ways that contradict those claims is waving a red flag. When actions and words don't match, *believe the actions.*

ADHD disclaimer: Sometimes it feels like we have to sell ourselves, right? Like if we don't point out our good qualities, people won't notice them. It's that anxious energy of, "Pick me! I promise I'm a good friend! Let me explain why!" Underneath it all is the fear that people won't see us clearly—or won't see us in a positive light—unless we convince them.

But here's the tricky part: Rather than build trust, this often does the opposite. It can actually make people doubt us, not because we're untrustworthy, but because trust is felt over time, not proven with words. In fact, what we intend as reassurance can sometimes come across as a red flag.

Think about it. Honest, loyal, and caring—fill in the blank—people don't go around declaring their honesty. They simply are. Trustworthy people don't need to announce their trustworthiness; they demonstrate it through consistent actions.

On the other hand, unsafe people tell you who they are instead of showing you, because words are easier to manipulate. Here's why they do it:

- *They want to control the narrative.* People without integrity often use words to shape how others perceive them. "I'm a really good friend" or "You can always trust me" allows them to dictate how they're seen.

- *They substitute action with words.* Unsafe people might say what you want to hear, knowing it creates a false sense of security. But words without follow-through are meaningless. If someone consistently reassures you of their loyalty while disregarding your boundaries or letting you down, their words are just smoke and mirrors.

- *They rely on charm over substance.* Manipulative people depend on charm, flattery, or big promises instead of consistently demonstrating respect and accountability.

- *They don't want to be questioned.* When someone repeatedly asserts their trustworthiness, it can be a defense mechanism. They might be consciously or unconsciously aware that their actions could raise doubts, so they overcompensate by reinforcing their verbal image.

- *They are avoiding accountability.* By proclaiming their identity, unsafe people can avoid self-reflection. If they constantly say "I'm a good person," they may feel no need to examine or change their harmful behavior.

If you grew up in an environment where words didn't align with actions, you might have learned to trust the words more than the behavior. But here's the thing: Safe people don't need to constantly remind you of their safety; you simply know it. Sure, safe people are still human and they'll make mistakes—but they'll take responsibility and work to repair things.

Unsafe people will keep talking. Your job is to stop listening and start watching. And for those of us with ADHD, it's a good reminder to stop trying to sell ourselves and start living our values. Trust grows from what we do—not what we explain.

Boundaries

Setting boundaries isn't about canceling, cutting off, or controlling others. It's about making choices that reflect self-respect while still maintaining healthy, reciprocal relationships.

Unhealthy and healthy boundaries might look similar at first glance, but the intention behind them makes all the difference. Unhealthy boundaries often come from a place of trying to change, control, or manipulate someone else. Healthy boundaries, however, are about managing *yourself*, your choices, and your environment in a way that aligns with your values and well-being.

Here's the difference:

- **Unhealthy boundary:** "I will not live with someone using drugs, so *you need to stop*, or I'll have to move out." (You're hoping they'll change to avoid leaving.)

- **Healthy boundary:** "I will not live in an environment where drug use is happening, so *if that continues*, I will move out." (You're setting your standard and acting in alignment with it, without trying to control them.)

In both cases, the action is the same—you're ready to move out if the drug use continues. But with the unhealthy boundary, you're hoping they'll change to avoid having to leave. With the healthy boundary, you recognize it's about protecting your own well-being and not manipulating the other person into compliance.

Here are some more examples:

Healthy Boundary (Managing Yourself)	Unhealthy Boundary (Managing Others)
If I'm spoken to disrespectfully, I will walk away.	*You need to stop talking to me like that.*
If I find content offensive, I will unfollow or block.	*You have to stop posting offensive content.*
If I'm yelled at, I will remove myself from the conversation.	*Please don't yell at me.*

Narcissistic Behavior and Abuse

Manipulative behavior is toxic, especially for neurodiverse people. Our executive functioning challenges make us more vulnerable to manipulation. We tend to feel deeply, empathize intensely, and crave meaningful connections. Manipulators, including narcissists, know this well: *If you can control people's feelings, you can control people.*

They often prey on our insecurities, making it easier to manipulate the narrative. For those struggling with self-trust, impulsiveness, and rejection sensitivity, these behaviors can be disorienting. Gaslighting and love bombing are common examples that leave you chasing approval and unsure of where the relationship truly stands.

Not every person who behaves this way is a narcissist. Some may simply lack emotional maturity, but the harm can still be real.

Let's look at how these behaviors work and how to protect yourself from them.

Gaslighting. *Gaslighting* is a manipulation tactic that makes you doubt your own perception, memory, or feelings. Here are some common tactics to watch for:

Twisting your words to make you question reality:

- "I never said that. You must have imagined it."

- "Your ADHD brain just forgot."

Blaming you for their behavior:

- "You made me yell at you. If you'd just listened…"

- "I wouldn't treat you this way if you weren't so difficult."

Dismissing your feelings and making you feel irrational:

- "You're overreacting. It's not a big deal."

- "Why do you always make everything about you?"

Using your ADHD against you:

- "Maybe it's just your ADHD making you too sensitive."

- "You always forget things and change your mind."

Denying past behavior:

- "That never happened. Stop making things up."

- "I only said that because I was joking. You take everything so seriously."

Making you feel like you're the problem:

- "Everyone else is fine with me. You're the only one who has an issue."

- "You need to work on your communication skills."

Creating dependency:

- "You'd be lost without me."

- "You're lucky I understand you."

Gaslighting, whether intentional or not, can make you doubt yourself. But there are ways to protect yourself:

- ☑ **Write it down.** Track conversations, events, and your feelings.

- ☑ **Trust your instincts.** If something feels off, don't dismiss your emotions.

- ☑ **Get a reality check.** Talk to trusted friends or a therapist.

- ☑ **Believe actions over words.** If someone's behavior contradicts their words, trust what you see.

- ☑ **Stop over-explaining.** You don't need to prove your reality to someone who refuses to see it.

- ☑ **Take space.** Emotional distance helps you see patterns more clearly.

- ☑ **Set boundaries.** If someone keeps making you doubt yourself, limit their influence.

- ☑ **Know the real issue.** ADHD may affect memory, but it doesn't excuse toxic behavior.

Spotting manipulation allows you to protect yourself and build relationships based on genuine trust—not control.

Love bombing. *Love bombing* happens when someone showers you with overwhelming affection, attention, or promises early on to quickly create trust and dependency. It feels exciting and validating, like you've finally found someone who really gets you.

But watch out! ADHDers tend to form strong emotional attachments quickly and can get hyperfocused on relationships, making us especially vulnerable to love bombing. It's like getting sucked into a flashy infomercial: "Act now! This love is unlike anything you've ever felt!"—only to realize later it's not as advertised, and now you're emotionally drained.

Our brains sometimes confuse feeling good with being good. If someone makes us feel special, we might assume they're trustworthy. This is emotional reasoning, where we believe something is true just because we feel it deeply. But feelings aren't facts, and an intense connection doesn't always mean a real one.

Love bombing can look like:

- Excessive praise and attention—"I've never met anyone like you: you're perfect"

- Fast-tracking commitment—"I just feel like we're meant to be"

- Grand gestures that feel like too much, too soon—lavish gifts, constant texting, wanting to spend all their time with you

- Creating dependency—they make you feel special, then pull back, making you chase their approval

ADHDers are vulnerable to love bombing, but we can also fall into this behavior. The difference between ADHDers and narcissists is the intention. ADHDers express affection early on because they're genuinely excited. For narcissists, the intensity is a setup. Once you're hooked, they flip the script, and you end up walking on eggshells, trying to regain their affection.

Narcissists use love bombing to gain control, not build a real connection. Their goal is to make you dependent on them. To protect yourself, slow things down and let trust build over time.

Here's how to pace things:

- For friendships, observe their behavior for three to six months before opening up deeply.

- For romantic relationships, trust and intimacy should develop over six months to a year.

Pay attention to how they handle conflict and treat others. Safe people respect differences, while unsafe people react with blame. And remember, trust is built through consistent behavior, not one grand gesture.

Future faking. *Future faking* is when someone makes big promises about what they'll do—"We'll travel the world!" "I'll change!" "You're the one I'll marry someday"—with no real plan to follow through. The goal isn't to build a future but to keep you hooked. ADHDers, who are hopeful and tend to focus on what could be, are especially at risk. If someone's words feel amazing but their actions don't match, hit pause. Real connection is built on what they do, not just what they say.

When it's abuse. It's one thing to tolerate harmless quirks, everyday frustrations, and the occasional bad mood. That's part of being in relationships with real, imperfect humans. But tolerating harmful or abusive behavior? That's a whole different story.

Safe people might mess up, but they won't make you feel small, powerless, or afraid. They take responsibility for their actions, apologize, and work to repair the damage.

Abuse isn't about having a bad day; it's a pattern of behavior designed to control, manipulate, or degrade. This can look like repeated boundary violations, gaslighting, blame-shifting, or emotional invalidation.

Sometimes, people act out of emotional immaturity. They may not mean to manipulate you, but their actions still hurt. Emotional immaturity can show up in manipulative behavior, where someone may not take responsibility or acknowledge how their actions affect you. Recognizing the difference between this and intentional abuse can be tricky, but it's important to distinguish between someone who's emotionally immature and someone who's actively manipulating.

If you're unsure whether someone's behavior is toxic or just a mistake, ask yourself:

- *Is this a one-time thing or a repeated pattern?*

- *When I express how I feel, do they take accountability or shift blame?*

- *Do I feel safe and valued in this relationship, or am I constantly walking on eggshells?*

- *Do they try to repair the damage, or dismiss my feelings?*

If something feels off, trust your gut. But if you're struggling to figure out what "off" even feels like, it might be because of ADHD or alexithymia (difficulty identifying emotions). If that's the case, try looking for patterns in behavior. Does this person's actions match their words? Do you feel drained or second-guess yourself when you are with them? If so, take that as information. You don't need to have a perfect explanation to justify your discomfort.

If in doubt, reach out! Seeking support, whether from a therapist, a trusted friend, or a support group, is not a weakness. It's self-respect.

Reclaiming Your Power

Social media is full of advice on self-care, boundaries, and emotional well-being. Some of it is helpful, but a lot of it is misleading and encouraging two extremes:

- Codependence disguised as empowerment—"If they don't validate you, cut them off. If they trigger you, they're toxic. If they don't meet your needs, they don't deserve a place in your life."

- Hyper-independence disguised as strength—"You don't need anyone. Relying on others is a weakness. Never explain yourself, never look back."

But neither of these leads to true well-being. One keeps you dependent on others for emotion regulation, while the other isolates you from the support you need.

The truth is, we thrive on *interdependence*, the ability to turn to others for support when needed, while also relying on our own internal resources when that support isn't available. This is emotional maturity. It's not about waiting for the world to accommodate you or rejecting connection entirely. It's understanding that while relationships help our well-being, they're not responsible for it.

Polyvagal theory tells us that co-regulation is a biological need, but it doesn't replace self-regulation. We need both! And that's where self-leadership comes in.

Self-Leadership

If your peace depends on getting others to act "correctly," you're always at their mercy. The world won't always meet your needs, and people won't always behave the way you want. You can't control what others think, feel, or do. But you can control how you respond.

Self-leadership means navigating life without relying on others to manage your emotional state. It's about shifting from external power (hoping others behave the right way) to internal power (knowing you can handle whatever comes your way). When you stop trying to control others and start managing yourself, you step into real power—the kind no one can take from you.

Triggers and Being "Canceled"

It might feel like emotional well-being comes from eliminating everything that triggers you. The idea that removing stressors will bring peace and that avoiding difficult situations means staying regulated sounds tempting. You might even hear advice like "If they upset you, cut them off" or "Go no-contact if they don't respect your boundaries."

But here's the catch—avoiding discomfort doesn't create strength. It just makes you dependent on external circumstances. If your strategy is to remove everything uncomfortable, you'll always feel fragile. If your peace depends on others behaving predictably, you'll always feel anxious. And if you expect others to change so you don't have to, you'll always feel powerless.

The real solution isn't about controlling what happens around you. It's about strengthening your ability to handle whatever life throws your way. Instead of asking *How can I avoid this trigger?* ask yourself:

- *How can I regulate myself when this happens?*

- *How do I handle discomfort without abandoning myself?*

- *What tools can I use to manage my response?*

- *What support systems help me stay grounded?*

- *How do I set boundaries that protect my well-being?*

- *How can I shift my perspective on this situation?*

The stronger your ability to self-regulate, the less power discomfort has over you. Situations that once sent you spiraling will eventually become things you can navigate with confidence.

This doesn't mean never avoiding harmful situations or relationships. Sometimes walking away is necessary. But remember, removing triggers from your life isn't the same as truly regulating your emotions.

And here's a thought: Sometimes discomfort isn't a sign to run. It's a sign to look deeper.

Think about earthworms after a heavy rain. You don't usually see them, but when the rain hits, they surface. The same is true for what's hidden inside. Triggers, stress, and emotional storms often bring up what we've buried. If you avoid every storm, you might never discover what needs healing.

Real power isn't about controlling who stays or goes in your life. It's about knowing how to manage what's happening right now and using it as an opportunity to grow.

Conclusion

ADHD often makes us see the best in others and hope for the best in every situation. But this openness can also leave us vulnerable to being taken advantage of. The good news is that you can start to choose who you allow into your life and how much influence they have over you. You don't have to believe everything others say, especially when it doesn't feel right.

Throughout this chapter, you've learned to recognize harmful feedback, understand who's safe, and set boundaries. For too long, you might have been told you can't trust yourself. But now, you can start to correct that. You have the power to trust your instincts, make decisions based on what feels true for you, and reclaim your personal strength.

You have the power to lead yourself. By trusting yourself and your choices, you'll navigate relationships with confidence, setting the tone for healthier connections. No longer will your worth be tested or defined by others—you'll create relationships where you can thrive as your true self.

A Closing Letter

You did it, brave soul! Congratulations!

This may be the final chapter, but it's not the end of your journey. You've spent your life navigating a world that wasn't built for your brain. Along the way, you've taken on criticism disguised as advice, internalized blame and shame that wasn't yours, and struggled to trust your own perceptions, especially when others dismissed them.

Here's the truth: You don't need the world to "get it right" for you to be alright. Life is messy, people make mistakes, and being human isn't easy. But you can find joy and peace in your own way.

I hope this book has helped you decode your nervous system; recognize your vulnerabilities; manage your emotions, energy, and time; and navigate relationships shame-free. You've learned to communicate effectively, attune with others, discern feedback, identify safe and unsafe people, and set boundaries that honor your needs without trying to control others. Most important, you've learned that true power doesn't come from managing the world around you; it comes from leading yourself.

Even with all the skills you've gained, relationships will still present challenges. Misunderstandings will happen, people will overstep your boundaries, and things won't always go smoothly. But now you have a new way of responding—a way that honors your values. You can pause and assess instead of absorbing blame and shame. You can act with integrity instead of tolerating mistreatment. You can validate yourself, instead of waiting for others to do it for you.

I'm so proud of you for pressing on, stepping outside your comfort zone, and daring to believe that you could do something amazing. As I always say, we're exceptionally good at doing the impossible!

Remember, you can rewire your nervous system. With practice, you can reshape how your body responds to the world around you. Keep revisiting the content—it's a lot to absorb. And don't forget to check out the bonus materials (http://www.newharbinger.com/56166) to support your learning.

Thank you for taking this journey with me. I'm cheering you on every step of the way. Wishing you all the success in the world!

Warmly,

Dr. Shawn

PS: I would love to hear from you. You can send a message on the website at http://www.drshawnhorn.com.

Acknowledgments

Writing this book has been a journey of learning, growth, and deep gratitude. I couldn't have done it alone and am thankful to the many people who supported and inspired me along the way.

To my family—Joel, Jacob, Bre, Sarah, Andrew, Paul and Sally Ayer, Diann and T.J. Knowles, Eldon and Meri Horn, and Deann Ayer—your love and support have been my foundation. Thank you for lifting me up and reminding me what matters most.

To my literary agent, Keely Boeving—your guidance and belief in this project helped bring it to life.

To my editors—Beth Bolton, Elizabeth Hollis Hansen, Joyce Wu, Jennye Garibaldi, Mary Gentile, and Atlas and Avery Griffin—thank you for your keen insights and care in shaping this work.

To New Harbinger Publications, Matthew McKay, and Tesilya Hanauer—thank you for believing in this book and giving it a home.

To my assistant, Brooklyn Graham—thank you for keeping everything moving smoothly and being a steady presence throughout this process.

To my office mate, Rich Wilson—thank you for walking this professional journey with me and always supporting my dreams.

To Dr. Zoe Shaw—your encouragement and generosity opened doors I never imagined. I'm deeply grateful for your support.

To the thought leaders who've shaped my work—Stephen Porges, Deb Dana, Russell Barkley, William W. Dodson, John Bradshaw, Marsha Linehan, John and Julie Gottman, and Stephanie Moulton Sarkis—thank you for your groundbreaking contributions.

To my clients—thank you for your support, patience, and inspiration as I wrote this book.

To my YouTube audience—your incredible response sparked this project and gave it life.

And to every reader holding this book—thank you for your curiosity, openness, and courage. This book is for you.

With deep gratitude,

Shawn Horn, PsyD

References

Alt, Mary, and Michelle L. Gutman. 2009. "Fast Mapping Semantic Features: Performance of Adults with Normal Language, History of Disorders of Spoken and Written Language, and Attention Deficit Hyperactivity Disorder on a Word-Learning Task." *Journal of Communication Disorders* 42, no. 5: 347–64. https://doi.org/10.1016/j.jcomdis.2009.03.004.

American Psychiatric Association. 2022. *Diagnostic and Statistical Manual of Mental Disorders, Fifth edition, Text Revision* (DSM-5-TR). Washington, DC: APA Publishing.

Arnsten, Amy FT. 2009. "The Emerging Neurobiology of Attention Deficit Hyperactivity Disorder: The Key Role of the Prefrontal Association Cortex." *The Journal of Pediatrics* 154, no. 5: I–S43.

Barkley, Russell A. 1997. *ADHD and the Nature of Self-Control.* New York: Guilford Press.

Barkley, Russell A. 2012. *Executive Functions: What They Are, How They Work, and Why They Evolved.* New York: Guilford Press.

Brach, Tara. 2019. *Radical Compassion: Learning to Love Yourself and Your World with the Practice of RAIN.* New York: Viking.

Bradshaw, John. 1988. *Healing the Shame That Binds You.* Health Communications.

Dana, Deb. 2018. *The Polyvagal Theory in Therapy: Engaging the Rhythm of Regulation.* New York: W. W. Norton & Company.

Dodson, William W. "Rejection Can Be More Painful with ADHD." *CHADD (Children and Adults with Attention-Deficit/Hyperactivity Disorder), ADHD Weekly,* April 4, 2019. https://chadd.org/adhd-weekly/rejection-can-more-painful-with-adhd/.

Goleman, Daniel, and Richard Davidson. 2017. *Altered Traits: Science Reveals How Meditation Changes Your Mind, Brain, and Body.* New York: Avery.

Gottman, John M., and Julie Schwartz Gottman. 2018. *The Science of Couples and Family Therapy: Behind the Scenes at the "Love Lab."* W. W. Norton & Company.

Guiard, Yves, and Olivier Rioul. 2015. "A Mathematical Description of the Speed/Accuracy Trade-Off of Aimed Movement." *Proceedings of the 2015 British HCI Conference*, 91–100. New York: ACM Press. https://doi.org/10.1145/2783446.2783574.

Huth, Alexander G., Wendy A. de Heer, Thomas L. Griffiths, Frédéric E. Theunissen, and Jack L. Gallant. 2016. "Natural Speech Reveals the Semantic Maps That Tile Human Cerebral Cortex." *Nature* 532: 453–458.

Lewis, Michael. 1995. *Shame: The Exposed Self.* New York: The Free Press.

Lewis, Michael. 2022. "The Self-Conscious Emotions." *Encyclopedia on Early Childhood Development.* https://www.child-encyclopedia.com/emotions/according-experts/self-conscious-emotions.

Miller, George A. 1956. "The Magical Number Seven, Plus or Minus Two: Some Limits on Our Capacity for Processing Information." *Psychological Review* 63, no. 2: 81–97.

Neff, Kristin. 2011. *Self-Compassion: The Proven Power of Being Kind to Yourself.* New York: William Morrow.

Nikkelen, S. W. C., P. M. Valkenburg, M. Huizinga, and B.J. Bushman. 2014. Media use and ADHD-related behaviors in children and adolescents: A meta-analysis. *Developmental Psychology*, 50 no. 9, 2228–2241. https://doi.org/10.1037/a0037318

Porges, Stephen W. 2011. *The Polyvagal Theory: Neurophysiological Foundations of Emotions, Attachment, Communication, and Self-Regulation.* New York: W. W. Norton & Company.

Pritchard, Alison E., Carly A. Nigro, Lisa A. Jacobson, and Mark E. Mahone. 2012. "The Role of Neuropsychological Assessment in the Functional Outcomes of Children with ADHD." *Neuropsychology Review* 22, no. 1: 54–68. https://doi.org/10.1007/s11065-011-9185-7.

Shaw, Philip, Argyris Stringaris, Joel Nigg, and Ellen Leibenluft. 2014. "Emotion Dysregulation in Attention Deficit Hyperactivity Disorder." *American Journal of Psychiatry* 171, no. 3: 276–293.

Volkow, Nora D., Gene-Jack Wang, Scott H. Kollins, Tim L. Wigal, Jeffrey H. Newcorn, Frank Telang, et al. 2009. "Evaluating Dopamine Reward Pathway in ADHD: Clinical Implications." *JAMA* 302, no. 10: 1084–1091. doi:10.1001/jama.2009.1308

Shawn Horn, PsyD, is a licensed clinical psychologist, keynote and TEDx speaker, and author with over three decades of experience in the mental health field. She specializes in providing psychotherapy for adults with attention-deficit/hyperactivity disorder (ADHD), with a focus on shame resilience, polyvagal-informed nervous system regulation, and emotion regulation.

In addition to her private practice, Horn has served as adjunct faculty at Gonzaga University and Moody Bible Seminary, and as a psychotherapy supervisor for the University of Washington and Washington State-affiliated psychiatric residency program in Spokane, WA. Known as the "Shame-Busting Psychologist" on social media, she reaches thousands with her honest and informative content on adult ADHD, rejection sensitive dysphoria (RSD), and mental health education. She is also the host of the *Inspired Living* podcast and blog, where she brings her expertise and encouragement to a wider audience.

Foreword writer **Stephanie Moulton Sarkis, PhD,** is a psychotherapist specializing in ADHD, anxiety, and narcissistic abuse. She is author of eight books and three workbooks, including *Gaslighting: Recognize Manipulative and Emotionally Abusive People—and Break Free* and *Healing from Toxic Relationships*. Sarkis has been in private practice for more than twenty-five years, and hosts the *Talking Brains* podcast. She is based in Tampa, FL. Learn more at www.stephaniesarkis.com.

Real change *is* possible

For more than fifty years, New Harbinger has published proven-effective self-help books and pioneering workbooks to help readers of all ages and backgrounds improve mental health and well-being, and achieve lasting personal growth. In addition, our spirituality books offer profound guidance for deepening awareness and cultivating healing, self-discovery, and fulfillment.

Founded by psychologist Matthew McKay and Patrick Fanning, New Harbinger is proud to be an independent, employee-owned company. Our books reflect our core values of integrity, innovation, commitment, sustainability, compassion, and trust. Written by leaders in the field and recommended by therapists worldwide, New Harbinger books are practical, accessible, and provide real tools for real change.

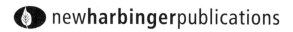 **newharbinger**publications

MORE BOOKS from
NEW HARBINGER PUBLICATIONS

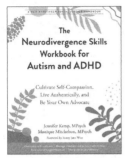
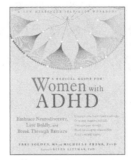
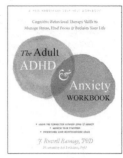
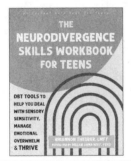
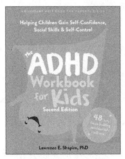
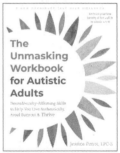

Did you know there are **free tools** you can download for this book?

Free tools are things like **worksheets, guided meditation exercises**, and **more** that will help you get the most out of your book.

You can download free tools for this book— whether you bought or borrowed it, in any format, from any source—from the New Harbinger website. All you need is a NewHarbinger.com account. Just use the URL provided in this book to view the free tools that are available for it. Then, click on the "download" button for the free tool you want, and follow the prompts that appear to log in to your NewHarbinger.com account and download the material.

You can also save the free tools for this book to your **Free Tools Library** so you can access them again anytime, just by logging in to your account! Just look for this button on the book's free tools page.

+ Save this to my free tools library

If you need help accessing or downloading free tools, visit **newharbinger.com/faq** or contact us at **customerservice@newharbinger.com**.